Underlying Standards that Support Population Health Improvement

Underlying Standards that Support Population Health Improvement

Laura Bright • Johanna Goderre

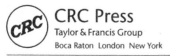

CRC Press
Taylor & Francis Group
Boca Raton London New York

CRC Press is an imprint of the
Taylor & Francis Group, an **informa** business
A PRODUCTIVITY PRESS BOOK

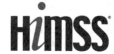

CRC Press
Taylor & Francis Group
6000 Broken Sound Parkway NW, Suite 300
Boca Raton, FL 33487-2742

First issued in paperback 2022

© 2018 by Taylor & Francis Group, LLC <change as necessary>
CRC Press is an imprint of Taylor & Francis Group, an Informa business

No claim to original U.S. Government works

ISBN-13: 978-1-498-76145-1 (hbk)
ISBN-13: 978-1-03-233940-5 (pbk)
DOI: 10.4324/9781315153230

Publisher's Note

The publisher has gone to great lengths to ensure the quality of this reprint but points out that some imperfections in the original copies may be apparent.

Visit the Taylor & Francis Web site at
http://www.taylorandfrancis.com

and the CRC Press Web site at
http://www.crcpress.com

Contents

Preface

The editors of this book came into the field of standards development and implementation in very different ways. Laura entered the healthcare standards world from the standpoint of a software developer and systems architect, two fields where the value of standard representations of data and communications protocols are well understood; indeed, nothing in software works without them. From Johanna's perspective in public health, her stakeholders had a much harder time understanding the benefits a standards-based approach to their projects would bring, in large part because the standards themselves are too often difficult to understand. This is an all-too-common problem in the healthcare standards space; the writers of the standards are very technically focused people, and they write in very technical ways, which leaves the users and implementers saying, "Why do I need to do all this? Why does it have to be so complicated?"

With this book, we hope to address both of those questions by highlighting success stories in implementing health IT standards in clear and easy terms. Each chapter relates a case study demonstrating how standards further interoperable health data exchange, especially in the service of advancing tools to monitor population health and public health. These are stories that demonstrate how bringing the right stakeholders together on standards-based projects can bridge divides between software architects and clinical end users, health system decision-makers, and standards authors.

Our first chapter begins with an overview of the history of standards, delving into what exactly we mean by a standard, where the concept of standards started, and how we got where we are today. It gives a nontechnical view into the software and standards architect's perspective on the necessary components of successful implementations to better explain the "why" behind standards, the testing of standards, and how to ensure better end-user experiences.

Our first case study in Chapter 2 looks at early childhood public health, and the process behind the early detection of hearing problems in newborns. The state of Oregon has implemented the IHE Quality, Research, and Public Health (QRPH) Early Hearing Detection and Intervention (EHDI) Profile to receive live newborn hearing screening results electronically from a partner hospital's electronic health records (EHRs) system. The project was intended to reduce duplicative data entry for hospital screening partners and improve the timeliness, completeness, and quality of the newborn hearing screening data received, and has had very positive results.

From Oregon we move on to the Veneto region of Italy, and the Regions of Europe Working Together for Health (RENEWING HEALTH) project, whose focus is the use of integrated telemedicine services in the monitoring of chronic patients suffering from cardiovascular disease, chronic obstructive pulmonary disease, and diabetes. The use of telemonitoring services allows for more effective management of chronic patients by ensuring the continuity of care between the various clinical figures, allowing clinicians to have a constantly updated clinical status of their patients.

Immunizations are a critical tool for the protection of public health and are the focus of Chapter 4. Immunization information systems (IISs) and immunization registries have become invaluable tools for tracking immunization rates, tracking vaccine availability, and ensuring that children get all of the immunizations they need. For years, IISs have collected, analyzed, and reported on immunization-related data across the United States. This chapter examines how the use of standards and consistent methods of data capture for immunizations improve both individual health and public health by providing more accurate and timely data on rates of immunizations, reducing precautionary vaccinations, managing inventories and programs, and identifying populations at risk.

Our next venture into standards takes us to the Bumrungrad International Hospital in Bangkok, Thailand, which treats over 1.1 million patients annually from 190 countries. Bumrungrad International Hospital has a patient population that presents some unique challenges. A high proportion of the patients treated in the facility are from other countries, and to treat them, medical records must be coordinated globally and from a variety of national health infrastructures. Bumrungrad International Hospital has adapted the IHE Patient Plan of Care profile, which describes a standard way of exchanging nursing data and care plans for patients. This chapter describes the process used by Bumrungrad to adopt this standard for care planning in the clinical environment, the interoperability challenges faced, and the solutions developed by the site.

Diagnostic imaging and radiology have been a vital part of healthcare for many years, but much more recent is the idea that having access to images can be of benefit to all clinicians, not just those in the radiology department. eHealth Ontario, an independent agency of the Ontario Ministry of Health and Long-Term Care, developed a standards-based system called the Diagnostic Imaging Common Service (DI CS). DI CS enables the sharing and viewing of patients' diagnostic images and reports from across Ontario to hospital- and community-based healthcare providers anytime, anywhere. Chapter 6 takes a look at the DI CS system, including the standards used and related supporting systems, as well as the provincial approach to governance and data best practices.

The final three chapters deal with vital records (VR): a program most nations have to track life events such as births, deaths, and marriages. Across the United States, state departments of health VR programs are modernizing their information systems with the use of e-vital records—the electronic exchange of VR information between EHRs and state VR systems. Over the past several years, the National Center for Health Statistics (NCHS) has collaborated with the National Association for Public Health Statistics and Information Systems (NAPHSIS), EHR and VR system vendors, and other VR stakeholders to create standards for the exchange, sharing, and retrieval of information required for birth, death, and fetal death reporting. Chapter 7 takes us through the process used by NCHS to develop the standards required, while Chapters 8 and 9 describe projects by individual states to implement the standards that were developed. Chapter 8 introduces a project by the state of Minnesota to make their birth reporting electronic. Chapter 9 explores the other end of VR and the death reporting system developed by the state of Utah.

Our goal in creating this book is to give you, the users, clinicians, and administrators of the healthcare system, a better understanding of why standards exist and maybe spark some ideas for how standards might be able to improve your own projects. We hope you find it useful.

Laura Bright and Johanna Goderre

Acknowledgments

This work was funded by the Centers for Disease Prevention and Control, National Center for Health Statistics through the Vital Statistics Cooperative Program—Special Projects #200-2012-50824 Task Order 0002.

Editors

Laura Bright is a health informatics and standards consultant based in Toronto, Canada. She is currently the cochair of the Quality, Research, and Public Health Planning Committee at IHE, is a past cochair of the Patient Care Coordination Technical Committee, and has also been a member and the secretariat of the IHE Canada Steering Committee and a board member and director-at-large of IHE Canada. She is a strong advocate of ensuring a broad and international perspective on standards authorship. Laura has also recently been active in developing standards for privacy and security, clinical documents, and care delivery.

Laura's 18-year career in healthcare covers a wide variety of disciplines, including experience in planning, developing, and implementing innovative health IT solutions in a variety of environments. Notable projects include the development of treatment-planning software for stereotactic radiation therapy, an innovative project to produce software for both image-guided and imageless hip and knee replacement surgery, and the development of an eMPI, nonoperational data repositories, an EHR viewer, and patient portals. During this period, Laura also obtained her project management professional credentials and CPHIMS/CPHIMS-CA certifications. In recent years, she has contributed her expertise and experience as a senior architect, product manager, and standards specialist both in the private and public sectors, most recently serving as a diagnostic imaging subject matter expert for the Kingdom of Saudi Arabia Ministry of Health.

Johanna Goderre is a public health professional with over 10 years' experience conducting public health studies, from concept development and grant application to implementation, quality assurance, analysis, and publication in an academic research setting. Her professional experience and interests bridge technical domains such as IT and statistical analysis with health domains that deliver high-quality, evidenced-based care to large populations, thus ensuring these often separate worlds can come together to use their own data to advance health improvements.

Johanna came to the standards world through a project to develop family planning standards in two IHE committees: Information Technology Infrastructure and Quality, Research, and Public Health. These standards will support transitioning an aggregate service delivery reporting system to a twenty-first century encounter-level system that can return clinically relevant performance measures in a user-friendly and visually actionable manner. This new system will accept standards-based summaries of health encounters from EHR systems in over 4000 clinical settings in all US states and territories. In 15 months, she has been able to take a relatively little-known clinical field with few affiliations to health IT standards through the initial authorship of data exchange and clinical decision support standards to pilot testing, all with the clinical end users engaged in technical and privacy and security guidance.

Previously the senior health informatics advisor to the Office of Population Affairs in the US Department of Health and Human Services' Office of the Assistant Secretary for Health, Johanna is currently a senior consultant with the CedarBridge Group, LLC.

Chapter 1

Introduction: Standards and Health IT

Tone Southerland

Contents

Standards and Health IT

What Is a Standard Anyway?

According to the International Organization for Standardization (ISO), "A standard is a document that provides requirements, specifications, guidelines or characteristics that can be used consistently to ensure that materials, products, processes and services are fit for their purpose." However, this is not exactly what standardization has always meant; it has differed in form depending on setting and purpose. Standardization dates back to the beginning of time, being key in forming civilizations, allowing various nations and peoples to converge on approaches to farming, military strategies, roads, currencies, measurements, public health, and other areas in the interest of their survival.* Standardization was not optional if these civilizations were to not only survive but ultimately thrive and grow in wealth, knowledge, and influence.

While standards can be traced back several thousand years to developments such as currency and road building, it was not until the Industrial Revolution, which arguably started in the 1770s and ran into the 1830s, that the use of standards began to increase in a significant way. This was a major turning point in history for improving the lives of masses of people all across the world. It was also a key initiator of what we understand today as formal standardization. Although standardization certainly existed across all areas of life prior to this time, it began to take on a more formal approach during this era out of the necessity of managing the growth of various industries across the globe. Industries such as rail and steel and those that were driven by the development of the steam engine created new opportunities not only within various countries but also across international borders. When quality materials could not be obtained locally, they would be sourced from another country, oftentimes resulting in much higher costs that would be passed down to consumers. This problem encouraged producers to find ways to lower their prices, and these producers found that by instituting agreements between buyers and sellers of various materials that required the materials to be produced to a certain specification, this ultimately resulted in higher quality material for a better price. These benefits could be passed along to their customers, resulting in a greater volume of sales at significantly lower prices.†

Specific to the American experience was the case of rail manufacturing, where higher quality rail could be acquired from England; however, it was also substantially more expensive. Purchasers of American-made rail would create very specific work orders for those producing the rails in England to ensure the product they received was of high enough quality. Testing tools were even developed to ensure the quality of these rails. These testing tools were custom designed for specific situations and for specific versions of the materials being produced; each end product was put through unique testing. Modern-day testing tools, however, are designed to test many different

---

* http://www.iso.org/iso/home/standards.htm.
† *ASTM 1898–1998: A Century of Progress*. West Conshohocken, PA: ASTM, 1998.

products looking to achieve conformance or certification in a specific market or industry space.

The development and use of railway testing tools led to new understandings about the properties of the metals being used in the rails. Eventually, this led to the realization that the data collected from testing could feed into the creation of standards, resulting in a better situation for everyone involved. The result of these efforts was the creation of the American Society for Testing and Materials (ASTM) in 1898, and as they say, the rest is history.* Fast-forward more than 100 years and one will find that ASTM, in conjunction with Health Level Seven International (HL7), created the "Continuity of Care Document" (CCD)† implementation guide, which has become the backbone of content standardization in the medical record space. This signifies the ongoing development of new standards over time in order to continue to meet consumer needs for higher quality products at reasonable costs.

Businesses will always have a pressing need for their own standards that solve immediate problems related to ensuring quality products; however, this approach does not support standardization across entire industries to provide more choices to consumers and business partners. Standards are created either intentionally or unintentionally. That is, they are created for a specific purpose by an interested society that could be a government, a standards development organization (SDO), or some other group; or they are created without intention as a result of market forces providing the impetus for the broad success of a particular way of accomplishing something.‡ Within the intentional realm of creating standards we see, in the context of this text, that there are a couple of ways that this can be accomplished: (1) a government can implement a regulation and require significant numbers of businesses to comply, or (2) a volunteer-led society or consortium can be created requiring the buy-in of enough industry stakeholders to drive forward the creation of the standard. Either approach has the same end in mind: to have the majority, if not all, of the stakeholders in a particular society converge around following the same rules for creating products and services. While the latter is typically a better approach, as it is driven by market needs and not government mandates, the two approaches are often leveraged together in the interest of more efficiently and effectively driving forward market changes while minimizing production costs.

---

* *ASTM 1898–1998: A Century of Progress.* West Conshohocken, PA: ASTM, 1998.
† https://www.hl7.org/implement/standards/product_brief.cfm?product_id=6.
‡ http://www.sis.pitt.edu/spring/cgi-bin/mbsblogger.cgi?type=%5C2010%5C02%5Cstandproc.txt.

Community-led initiatives were created as a result of businesses realizing the value of standard approaches to some particular business activity. Two organizations would create an agreement between their companies that supported some mutual business interest. This would be expanded to include other organizations, and as a result, a community-based standard would be created. Many of these initial standards were created merely as by-products of business activities, not as intentional standards development activities. As time moved on, standards were scaled up and across industries when they made the work of some activity more efficient and the end result was of higher quality. The collaboration across so many organizations eventually led to a multi-stakeholder environment where many organizations came together to influence the standards for both the good of the industry as well as for specific practices that the participating organizations may have previously invested in developing.

One example of a joint approach involving multiple stakeholders in recent years is the creation of the Nationwide Health Information Network (NHIN) in the United States. This initiative was initially only available to participants that received their funding through US federal government grants. Later, the program evolved to include vendors operating outside of the public-funding realm, resulting in a boom in the number of participants. Today, this is known as the Sequoia Project eHealth Exchange Participant Testing Program. The Sequoia Project itself is governed by a coordinating committee consisting of representatives from many different organizations. The standards this program utilizes are published primarily out of Integrating the Healthcare Enterprise (IHE) and HL7. In addition, both IHE and HL7 are multi-stakeholder organizations in their own right, representing a very broad swath of the healthcare and information technology–based companies across the world.*

How is this history of standardization and the healthcare domain relevant to the role of a software architect in healthcare? Understanding the domain in which a software developer operates is very much needed to write software that is effective for end users. If one does not comprehend the basics of the field in which they need to operate, then they will not be able to understand the experience from the users' perspective, and thus will be likely to build a solution that might appear great in design but will perform poorly in actual use. The concept of domain-driven design was first introduced in 2003 by Eric Evans in his book of the same title, and Evans

---

* http://sequoiaproject.org/ehealth-exchange.

directly addresses this challenge by exploring the concept of creating models in software based specifically on use cases found within the domain in which they operate. Most, if not all, standards development organizations begin their work by identifying and developing use cases that describe specific steps taken within a scenario or set of scenarios that a customer or industry is focused on. These use cases feed into functional requirements that in turn drive the technical requirements, the sum of all of these parts resulting in the creation of the standard specification itself. Understanding that the world of health information technology (health IT) is driven strongly by formal standards as well as by the market is key to being successful in this space. By studying not only the standards themselves but also peeling back the proverbial onion to better understand the processes used to develop the standards provides for a great deal more insight into why certain decisions are made in health IT standards. This in turn provides software architects with the necessary insight to drive their designs to a place of success for their end users.

Software Engineering: From There to Here

The concept of machines doing physical work in place of humans dates back thousands of years; however, the concept of machines doing mental work of the same dates back only a few hundred years, beginning with Charles Babbage and Ada Lovelace, leading up to and beyond the invention of digital computers in the Alan Turing and John Atanasoff era. In order to expand the opportunities for digital computers to deliver on the promises of their ancestors, a new paradigm was needed to provide the opportunity for computers to scale to meet societal needs. This paradigm arrived in the form of computer programs that are built from developing software. The domain in which software is created is known as *software engineering*. According to Merriam-Webster, software engineering is defined as "a branch of computer science that deals with the design, implementation, and maintenance of complex computer programs."* The Institute of Electrical and Electronics Engineers (IEEE), the main society for engineers, refines this definition of software engineering to "the application of a systematic, disciplined, quantifiable approach to the design, development, operation, and maintenance of software, and the study of these approaches; that is, the application of

---

* http://www.merriam-webster.com/dictionary/software%20engineering.

engineering to software."* Regardless of which definition one might align more closely with, it is well known that the discipline of software engineering is critical to the current and future success of most, if not all, business domains.

As advancements in software were made, initially with the creation of languages such as Fortran, COBOL, and LISP in the 1950s, and then later with the development of parallel processing technologies allowing for software programs to be written and executed in more efficient ways, there became a need to manage the sheer volume of code that was being written by programmers. Solutions to address these problems arose as software programming paradigms and software development methodologies. Paradigms addressed the problem from the perspective of how the code was written (e.g., object oriented, aspect oriented, procedural), whereas methodologies (e.g., Waterfall, Agile, Rational Unified Process) addressed the problem from the perspective of how the code was managed throughout the development life cycle. Similar to the market's need to standardize across many domains, the field of software engineering also had this same need, and it was addressed through the creation of these programming paradigms and software development methodologies. In both of these areas, many standards have been and continue to be published to provide value to the citizens of the software engineering universe.

While software development methodologies will go a long way to satisfy the needs of individual software vendors internally, they do not address the larger challenge of standardization across the many different vendor products on the market today. Thus, further guidance in the implementation of such software programs is quite important in regard to attaining widespread use of these software applications in the healthcare domain. This ensures that such systems can interact in ways that are reasonably attainable by both the vendors and end users alike.

Methodologies, Philosophies, and Complexity

The IT field continues to struggle with keeping projects on time, under budget, and meeting end-user expectations because it is ultimately a very difficult task to organize people as they create a large, complex project with many interconnected requirements. Over several decades, methodologies

---

* http://programmers.stackexchange.com/questions/183685/problem-understanding-the-ieee -definition-of-software-engineering.

such as Waterfall, Systems Development Life Cycle (SDLC), Rapid Application Development (RAD), Extreme Programming (XP), Agile, and others were developed in an attempt to curb the continual challenge of faulty software project estimations.

Software engineers are always trying to improve on their processes and find better ways to produce software and make code more manageable. The idea of *abstraction*, more concretely defined as *encapsulation*, which hides the details that one does not need to be fully aware of but still provides access to the functionality that those details support, is very much recursive in nature: once we abstract, or *black box*, a certain set of functionalities and publish them as a code library, that code library might then be packaged as part of another abstraction, and on the process goes as more and more complex systems are built. In conjunction with this focus on code reuse are efforts to build quality assurance automation tools to ensure any code dependencies remain functional through upgrades in either the source code library or the dependent code. In summary, this provides for a better implementation experience for the developer, and ultimately a better experience for the end user.

Given the complexity of today's IT world, an incremental or iterative approach must be used to secure an on-time and under-budget end result for almost any given IT project. A term often heard in the interoperability space of healthcare is *incremental interoperability*. This refers to the ability of a team crafting a product that has interoperable capabilities to gradually incorporate new functionality in very small pieces. Large interoperability code additions to an existing software product are a recipe for stalling almost any project, as the underlying standards are changing so rapidly that when the deployment of such a large code addition finally occurs, it is often grossly out of date and rendered mostly ineffective.

Even prior to the concept of incremental interoperability as we understand it today, in the 1990s, software engineers had a growing awareness that faster feedback mechanisms were needed in support of constantly changing requirements, and thus the *Agile Manifesto** was the birth of a new movement. Agile is based on four simple principles and may be implemented using a variety of tools. Specific decisions on how to go about implementing Agile are up to each individual organization, which at least in part is where it provides much of its value. Principally, there is a strong focus on the team aspect of building software; the first rule of the manifesto

---

* http://www.agilemanifesto.org.

is "Individuals and interactions over processes and tools." If we break this statement down we see that "and" is used, and not "or" in the conjunction of individuals and interactions. This is key: it is the combination of these two aspects that results in successful outcomes in projects. Additionally, in the *Agile Manifesto* is the "customer collaboration over contract negotiation" rule that signifies the importance of the relationship between the developer of the technology and the consumer or purchaser of the technology. Again, this circles back to this idea that solving problems in the IT field comes down to the people as much as it does the technology choices. In health IT, this is especially important as systems will never completely replace a clinician's ability to make certain judgment calls regarding patient care choices such as care plans, procedures, and other care guidance.

In my experience as a software architect and engineer in health IT, organizations that focus first on solving the business problems of customers and users are typically those that have more successful products—and happier customers and end users—while those organizations that focus on technology first struggle to satisfy end-user needs. This is not to say technology and standards choices are not important; they are certainly quite important, but priorities must be managed, and above all else, the business problem is what needs to be solved ahead of using a trendy tool or hot new technology.

I experienced this firsthand in a project I led during my time at Greenway Health (formerly Greenway Medical Technologies), centering around development for the Office of the National Coordinator for Health Information Technology's (ONC) 2014 Certification that supports centers for medicare and medicaid. I led the development team, working alongside a colleague who was leading the team of business analysts. We had a total of 19 people on our combined teams, 10 of whom I directed. We were notified by our internal leadership in November of 2012 that we would be the first electronic health record (EHR) vendor to certify for ONC 2014 Certification. Certification opened in early January 2013. This only allowed for about 8 weeks of development time. While we had completed some preparatory work leading up to this corporate decision of what we had to do by when, we still had our work cut out for us.

In the end, we were able to achieve our goal and became the first EHR vendor to certify under the new program. We were able to do this only by being very intentional with our communication at all points during the project, following Agile processes to ensure that any issues that were present were brought to the forefront immediately and dealt with accordingly.

Following our initial success, we then had to revise much of the functionality we developed to prepare it for deployment into production environments across our many customer sites. The next several months included a lot of communication not only between our internal teams but also between our business analyst team and our customers. The cornerstone of our ultimate success was the direct line of interaction with the clinicians using our product. This single aspect can be a huge factor in determining the success or failure of a software project.*

In the same vein, this is also relevant to the development of health IT standards, where interaction with end users is vital to producing standards and implementation guidance that matches what those end users need in order to administer care through the software they are using. As a software developer being tasked with creating standards-based functionality that also needs to meet the end-user expectations, it is important for the developer to think about two aspects of the workflows being addressed: (1) the functionality the end user is directly requesting and (2) the closest-matching workflow provided as guidance by the health IT standard. Sometimes these workflows do not align completely, and it becomes a vital task to identify the differences and understand their overall impact to the success of the project. For example, a workflow that a clinician user of a system follows will adhere to some protocol developed by a medical college, and this is typically great guidance. However, a health IT standard may have consulted with a different medical college or set of clinician experts, resulting in a slightly different workflow. Workflows may result in extra "clicks" in an application, or worse, a mismatch of information within the system, the latter of which might have grave consequences regarding the care of a patient.

In practice, I have experienced this quite often with health information exchange (HIE) implementations that are focused on meeting immediate end user needs and those priorities that their organizations set. The directors, managers, and end users that I work with rarely are concerned about the next version of any given standard that will be released unless it is one that will directly impact in a positive way the manner in which the end users of their solutions will use the system. This position is well justified as there are often significant budgetary constraints within which to work, and money spent toward solving a problem that might not ever be realized is a very real risk that must be avoided at all costs.

---

* http://www.ehrscope.com/blog/greenway-medical-prime-suite-ehr-first-to-receive-2014-onc-hit-certification.

Business Analysts Are the Secret Ingredient to Product Success

Problems that IT solutions unravel are done so not only by the technology itself and the way team members interact but also by the types of individuals that contribute to creating the product. Business analysts ensure that any functional requirements are well defined and as close as possible to what the customer expects the technology solution to deliver. They interact directly with key clinical personnel at provider organizations to feed into guidance around how clinical workflows need to be implemented in the product and in what priority. Business analysts act as a connection between end users and developers. They foster efficient and effective communication plans to ensure the workflows that clinicians need are represented properly in the final product.

In the healthcare industry business analysts also study health IT standards, changes in policy and regulation, and other initiatives that impact the solutions being developed. They delve into tomes of regulation for government incentive programs and translate their findings into business requirements that clinicians will need in their health IT solutions. The business analyst is a master in navigating translations between complex requirements, clinical workflows, and development efforts. As such, they are key to ensuring that solutions produced by vendors for end users are appropriately defined, customized, and implemented to meet the needs of those users.

Emerging Technical Solutions

APIs and Optionality

The field of software engineering is a craft. It requires thoughtfulness and creative approaches to solving problems. The software developer must consider which options he or she would like to leverage to solve the business problem being presented. This optionality is great in the right hands, but from a broader system interoperability perspective, such optionality must be constrained to further the integration opportunities of systems. The greater the amount of optionality that exists between any two interoperability products, the greater the chance that those two products will not align effectively out of the box. Project coordination becomes very important to ensure alignment is achieved, and this coordination takes time and costs money. As healthcare interoperability standards begin to mature (Digital Imaging and Communications in Medicine [DICOM] being one of the oldest, with an initial release date of 1985), they begin to be included more broadly in policy models such as state- and federal-level regulation. As long as this limits the amount of optionality, the resulting interoperability solution should provide valuable levels of usage to offset the cost of purchasing and installing the solutions.

One approach to optionality is through the use of an application programming interface (API), which provides an alternate way to interface with an external system. In its most basic form, an API is a way for IT systems or some sort of hardware component to interoperate, or interface, with another system or component to achieve some higher level of joint function or operation. The need to produce an API arises from a system's need to share a certain set of functionality with other systems, typically allowing end users to leverage the functionality of the other system as if it were in their own. APIs define requirements for transport, content, and security protocols and typically use common industry interoperability standards for this in the interest of achieving broad adoption levels. Many examples of APIs can be found in the industry today as the trend to interoperate in this manner is growing at a rapid pace.

In the context of information systems, and more specifically the Internet, APIs are typically seen in the form of *web APIs*—that is, APIs that are purpose-built to integrate functionality in web-based settings. Leveraging web-based technologies and environments means that a much broader level of adoption and integration is possible. More recently, EHR vendors have broached the API market by opening up their databases to provide easier access to the patient data needed for improving health outcomes for patients. Initiatives such as Substitutable Medical Apps, Reusable Technology (SMART) on Fast Healthcare Interoperability Resources (FHIR) are approaching the API space from the perspective of a marketplace, providing a platform where application vendors and EHR vendors can place their products that support an FHIR-based API technology stack. APIs support innovation by providing opportunities for new ideas to build into a specific niche in the market and by following a mash-up approach to building functionality where one particular product need not build (or rebuild) all the necessary functionality to achieve the end-user experience of the available product or service. The trend of APIs is ever increasing, and we will continue to see more of such opportunities in the future.

APIs also must account for security and authentication. Security is an important aspect of API integration that focuses on the encryption of data in motion—that is, data being exchanged between two systems. While

Transport Layer Security (TLS) is a well-defined, mostly well-understood, and typically well-implemented standard that is commonly used to secure data in motion, it is yet another layer that vendor solutions must be sure to account for in their overall offerings. With the increasing level of cyber security incidences being reported, this aspect of an API integration effort is becoming critical. Authentication is another very important concept for these vendors to understand and implement properly as well, as granting the wrong access to their systems can allow cyber security breaches, resulting in loss of data, the compromising of personal identities, and other issues. There are two parts to authentication: the authentication itself, which allows or dis-allows the user access, and the authorization of the user, which grants access to various parts of the system for a user that has been authenticated. The authentication portion is a binary approach, meaning the system connecting to the API either has access or does not have access. Authorization manages what level of access that system has—in other words, which transactions it can consume and what type and amount of data might be returned. For example, a 16-year-old motor vehicle operator in the state of Tennessee may be *authenticated* to operate a motor vehicle, but due to my license restrictions, I am only *authorized* to operate the vehicle during certain hours. My authorization level changes as I get older and acquire a new license with less restrictions. Computer systems work in much the same way around these concepts. There is an initial validation of whether or not a system user may gain access to a system, and then a subsequent check to see what level of access that user may be granted.

Today, authentication and authorization can be implemented a variety of ways, utilizing existing frameworks such as OAuth or WS-Security, or it may be achieved by developing a custom authentication framework. OAuth was created out of the efforts put forth by Twitter as they developed their API platform and is in broad use today. WS-Security was created as part of the W3C standards. Regardless of the technical solution selected for any given application, it is certainly a necessary piece to include in any product delivered to the customer. Additionally, we must also consider how we will manage the number of APIs that are expanding exponentially. According to ProgrammableWeb, there are over 16,000 APIs available today.* Since 2010, there has been a rough average growth rate of 27% per year of published APIs. At this rate, the industry will be at over 40,000 APIs by the year 2020. In 10 years? Almost 200,000. How are we going to

---

* http://www.programmableweb.com/api-research.

secure all of these APIs and ensure the end user has appropriate levels of security in their online experience? This is not a trivial problem to solve. A quick search on cyber security threats and reported incidents will give you a sense of the size of the issue. As more digital natives move into adulthood, the problem will only continue. We must persevere to find and implement appropriate policies and procedures to ensure users are safe-guarded, so that patients and clinicians alike will use software to improve health outcomes.

Projected API Growth

Year	No. of APIs
2016	16,000
2017	20,320
2018	25,806
2019	32,775
2020	41,623
2021	52,861
2022	67,133
2023	85,260
2024	108,280
2025	137,516
2026	174,645

APIs provide opportunities for consumers of information queries to deeply customize not only what information they pull back but also how they decide to go about using that information in their solutions. Some solutions may be provider focused (e.g., decision support, chronic disease management), whereas other solutions may be patient focused (e.g., access to longitudinal records, access to immunization information for children in public schools). Combining this flexibility with workflow-based implementation guidance provides a nice solution to the industry problem of scale regarding API platforms, as the flexibility inherent in APIs is still present to allow for continued growth and innovation in the industry, supporting diversified end users and solution sets.

Technologies such as artificial intelligence (AI) and natural language processing (NLP) attempt to deal with these sorts of problems by focusing a computer on interpreting text as if it were a human. Both AI and NLP are technologies that were expected to be much further along than they are to date. Both have been around for quite some time. AI entered around the same time computer research was getting heavy in the 1940s as part of Alan Turing's research. NLP was even prior to that, going back to the early 1900s in England, when the International Electrotechnical Commission (IEC) began the exploration of the use of terminologies to standardize parts that could be interchanged between different machines from the production line down to product delivery to bring higher value to those organizations purchasing such parts.

The development of AI technologies has not developed quite as fast or quite in the way that Turing anticipated it would. For example, Turing envisioned that computers would potentially replace people as companions, and I suppose they have to some extent, but not to any great extremes. People do not take their computers for walks in the parks or out to dinner; however, they are oftentimes fixated on their smartphones during these events. Computers have not supplanted the need for human interaction and connection.

There are many rubrics that can be applied in NLP algorithms, yet the value that NLP solutions bring often do not exceed the manpower required to create them in the first place. In other words, in many cases it would be better to not use any sort of NLP system at all. However, this does not mean that NLP does not have benefit and value in health IT and in the market in general. Much research is ongoing and progress is being slowly made. These aspects make this area of computer science one of the more complex and also one that has some of the highest potential to positively impact the use of health IT systems by clinicians and patients. Today, NLP is most relevant to working with the translation of narrative clinical notes into structured data that can be fed into decision support engines and used for other clinical guidance types of tools.

There are significant opportunities for advancement in health IT. However, these advancements will not arrive without overcoming challenges that exist today, such as those around scaling authorization across enterprises and abstracting away the complexities of solutions. There are certainly approaches such as abstraction that can help deal with these challenges, but it will ultimately be a combination of innovation, market drivers, and a broad adoption of standards that will lead to success.

Intersection of Software, Health IT, and Standards

Standards have been around in one form or another for centuries. Software, although certainly not as old, is developing its own history by producing patterns and innovations around what the next era of computers is shaping up to be. Health IT is a bit newer, being just a few decades old, and is arguably the last frontier of *electronification*. The next generation of clinicians will be digital natives, never knowing a day in their lives without technology being a part of not only their personal but also their professional lives. Many have asked why the standardization of healthcare in the IT sector is so hard; the reasons are many and could certainly be expounded on in their own tome. But to sum it up, it has to do with the human side of medical care, and that will never be fully converted over to being handled by a computer. There will always be a need for human assessment at some level; however, we do have much progress we can make yet around the standardization of health IT systems in the interest of significantly improving patient care and health outcomes.

In my own experience of developing health IT standards as well as implementing many of those same standards, standards developers must explore different options and achieve consensus for the mission of the standard, similar to the approach that software engineers might take when exploring their options for technical solutions to a specific business problem. Going through this process leaves one with a rather unique perspective on the standards development work processes and outcomes. Not only is there an appreciation for what has gone into the standards development work itself but also a much greater understanding of the *why*—that is, the reasoning and rationale behind creating the standard in the first place. Software engineers are known for answering questions with a simple yet sometimes frustrating phrase: "It depends." Why do they answer with this? Because clear and thorough explanations to many questions from business owners require a response representing a comprehensive perspective and critical thought applied to the solution. Without this, the solutions developed often do not meet the underlying business goals of the requester because assumptions made by a software engineer could be very different from those made from the business perspective. Seasoned software engineers have learned this and then follow with further questions to understand more. This is one perspective gained from participating in both the development of health IT standards and the implementation of those standards in products.

The importance of regulatory involvement in the development of health IT standards must not be underestimated. It is a combined effort of regulatory oversight and private industry innovations that will continue to drive forward the advancement of IT in the healthcare domain. As can be seen in the development of the Internet, the US federal government made a great deal of grant money available for universities to conduct research to create better ways to communicate with computer and telecommunication systems. While the US government desired a centrally controlled system, what they actually got was a decentralized system, which, as it turns out, was what the government really needed in the first place. A decentralized system provides built-in redundancy, as there is no single point of failure. What is particularly interesting about this is that by not exerting too much control over the specifics of the sponsored projects, the teams doing the work were allowed to think outside the box and create something leaning toward the larger societal interest. They were allowed to innovate. As software architects in health IT, we must also seek this same direction, finding opportunities to create our own unique solutions that will disrupt the status quo in how IT systems are used in healthcare today.

Policy, Payers, and Medical Records

Policy and regulatory guidance are required to push an industry forward that lacks the ability or circumstances to present the value statement to the stakeholders in a way that encourages forward movement without such government motivation. In other words, an industry that is "stuck," or challenged to move forward, because of shortsighted investors or broken economic models needs a boost to get over the hump, and regulatory incentives and requirements are a good source to move things along. Without the right level of government involvement and funding around the development of the first computers in the United States, there would have been a very different, and likely much later, development and use of computers. The government funded vast amounts of grants; upward of $6.5 million (2016 equivalent value) was spent to build the ENIAC alone, not to mention other federally funded projects that both preceded and succeeded that one.

This same type of situation is occurring in health IT now, as policy is being set from the federal government level with specific directions about what system developers must do to be compliant with the government mandates (e.g., Medicare Access and CHIP Reauthorization Act of 2015 and the

Quality Payment Program [MACRA/QPP]). However, the government has also learned to build in latitude with what they require and what the final deliverable will be from the system producers. More specifically, this is reflected in the choices of standards in the QPP regulation, many of which are still in their draft state. In addition, some of the requirements, such as that of EHR systems providing an API, are very loosely stated. It is smart on the side of the government to allow for continued innovation and growth in the private sector. As an architect in health IT, this is an important concept to grasp and should be leveraged to continue driving forward new ideas within your organization.

What's Next?

While the concept of software has been around for quite some time, the approaches to developing software have changed over time as the computers on which software is run change in their roles in business and society. As the use of computers has rapidly risen to become a part of almost every business and personal activity, the paradigms in which software developers must operate have also changed, oftentimes providing positive impact but sometimes not. On the front lines of software development, there is a continual search for better ways to accomplish the many complicated tasks that software development teams are responsible to deliver. This harkens back to the days of the Industrial Revolution, when testing tools were built to better understand the qualities of the steel being purchased for building railroads. While the context is certainly different in today's world, the reasoning and approach is more or less the same. Tools and products are built to create a better experience for software engineers, and in many cases, those tools drive the creation of standards.

Chapter 2

Early Hearing Detection and Intervention

Dina Dickerson, Meuy Swafford, and Heather Morrow-Almeida

Contents

Background

Early Hearing Detection and Intervention (EHDI) program staff are specialists such as otolaryngologists, public health nurses, and parents supporting parents in achieving three primary goals:

1. All infants are screened for hearing loss by 1 month of age.
2. Infants who do not pass newborn hearing screening receive diagnostic audiological services by 3 months of age.
3. Infants identified with hearing loss receive EHDI services by 6 months of age for optimal developmental outcomes.

In the United States, all 50 states and the District of Columbia have EHDI laws or voluntary compliance programs that support hearing screening for newborns.

In Oregon, all hospitals or birthing centers with more than 200 births per year are required to conduct newborn hearing screening within 1 month of the child's date of birth and report the results to the state EHDI program. Birth providers must also notify the newborn's parent or guardian as well as the healthcare provider of the screening results. Though not required to provide a newborn hearing screening by law, most small hospitals and many birth centers and midwives offer hearing screening as their standard of care. In Oregon, approximately 97% of all infants receive a newborn hearing screening.

The EHDI program of the Oregon Health Authority (OHA), the state-run health department, maintains a registry of all newborns and their hearing screening test results. Birthing facilities, including hospitals, birth centers, and independent midwives, report newborn hearing screening results using the Oregon Vital Events Registry System (OVERS). In addition to data elements collected on the birth certificate such as the child's name, date of birth, address, mother's name, mother's date of birth, telephone number, birth facility identifier, and newborn blood spot screening kit identifier, the screening facility must report the date of the screening, ear-specific results, and the type of equipment used, all within 10 days of completing the screening.

Collecting newborn hearing screening results through OVERS reduces the data entry burden for reporters, as only five additional screening-specific fields are required, in addition to the birth certificate data. Though making the reporting more manageable, data reporting through the birth certificate system is still duplicative, as the screening data are also entered in hospital electronic health records (EHRs).

There is still a need to reduce duplicative data entry and increase the timeliness and accuracy of screening result reporting to EHDI programs. Stakeholders from public health and health IT communities have developed technical specifications for data exchange between screening facilities' EHR systems and public health EHDI systems. Greater interoperability between clinical EHR systems and public health EHDI registries should help communities meet the hearing screening goals described previously and improve care coordination for deaf and hard of hearing (DHH) children. These interoperability specifications address how EHDI-related data can be exchanged between screening devices, EHRs used in birthing centers or pediatricians' offices, and systems used by audiologists or other specialists. Data can range from discrete readings from hearing screening devices to comprehensive plans describing the care needed for a DHH child. The adoption and use of these specifications is not widespread nationally; potential barriers may include EHDI programs' lack of familiarity with some of the technical concepts expressed and clinical partners' preoccupation with other technical challenges, including those related to federal EHR incentive programs and healthcare reform.

Objective

This chapter describes a pilot implementation of EHR interoperability specifications to improve newborn hearing screening reporting to OHA's EHDI registry. Funded by the Centers for Disease Control and Prevention (CDC)'s National Center for Birth Defects and Developmental Disabilities (NCBDDD) and the Office of Public Health Scientific Services (OPHSS), OHA partnered with the Oregon Health and Science University (OHSU), OZ Systems, Lantana Consulting, and the Public Health Informatics Institute (PHII) to conduct a pilot implementation of production hearing screening and care plan data exchange and to document the experience to inform future implementation and standards development.

The objective of the pilot was to implement the Integrating the Healthcare Enterprise (IHE) EHDI Profile interoperability specification allowing production screening data, meaning live patient data, sent by OHSU to be received as an electronic hearing plan of care (HPoC) document by OHA's EHDI program. Details on the implementation approach, partner roles, data exchange outcomes, and recommendations for other EHDI programs and future efforts in the development of interoperability standards follow.

Project Approach

In August 2014, funding was awarded to implement the Phase 2 pilot implementation of the IHE EHDI Profile for the exchange of production hearing screening and care plan data, with a project completion date of June 30, 2015. Phase 1 of this work did not involve actual patient data, while Phase 2 used live production data representing actual patients. A comparison of the Phase 1 and Phase 2 EHDI Clinical Document Architecture (CDA) pilots follows:

- Phase 1 occurred from 2012–2013 and was managed by the Public Health Data Standards Consortium (PHDSC). Activities in this phase were designed to simulate the process of reporting newborn hearing screening results from an EHR system to a state EHDI information system (EHDI-IS) registry. While the IHE "Early Hearing Care Plan" (EHCP) was written as a technical specification, it was first necessary to test the implementability of this specification in closer-to-real-life situations (or whatever reasoning is best). The primary goals of this testing included
  - Sending simulated newborn demographic and birth data in compliance with the EHDI Profile from an EHR system test harness
  - Using the Retrieve Form for Data Capture (RFD) specification* prepopulate demographic and birth data already known to the EHR system in a hearing screening results form
  - Receiving test data compliant with the EHDI Profile into the EHDI-IS test database
- Phase 2 occurred in 2014–2015 and was managed by PHII. This phase was designed to report production hearing screening results (meaning live patient data) from an EHR system to the state EHDI-IS registry. Lessons learned from Phase 1 were incorporated into a new version of the technical specification, renamed the IHE Profile HPoC. The goals of this phase included
  - Capturing live hearing screening results from an EHR system newborn assessment flow sheet

---

* http://www.ihe.net/Technical_Framework/upload/IHE_ITI_Suppl_RFD_Rev2-2_TI_2011-08-19.pdf.

- Sending newborn screening results from an EHR system using a Health Level Seven International (HL7) V2.*x* message and middleware vendor, where an HPoC was created based on decision support rules
- Sending the HPoC to the OHA system
- Demonstrating that the EHDI-IS live database could receive, parse, and consume the HPoC content from the EHR system

Partner Engagement

Once notified that Phase 2 was funded, it was necessary for all partners to reengage, review, and reestablish commitment to the project. The Oregon EHDI program staff reached out immediately to the project team and stakeholders, including OHSU audiologists and IT management and staff, in order to gauge their willingness to participate and their reception to a short timeline and limited funding. The full project team convened a kick-off call the last week of August 2014 to reaffirm commitments and to begin to define the project scope, establish a timeline, develop the work plan, and initiate the necessary contractual arrangements. This process is key to any health IT standards project to ensure that organizational roles and responsibilities are clearly defined.

The project role of each partner organization, including their part in supporting the IHE EHDI Profile, is described in Table 2.1.

Project Scope

The IHE EHDI Profile describes how hearing screening data can be sent from a screening device or EHR and converted into an electronic HPoC that can then be shared with the primary care providers and audiologists responsible for assuring timely diagnostic audiological evaluations to rule out hearing loss. The IHE EHDI Profile uses health information interoperability standards developed by HL7 and other standards development organizations.

Figure 2.1 illustrates the two main options for implementing the IHE EHDI Profile, both of which are described using technical terms that may be more familiar to health IT developers than public health practitioners. The first option calls for a Device Observation Reporter (e.g., a hearing screening device) to send results to a Device Observation Consumer and Content Creator (i.e., a related application such as an EHR), which generates a HPoC and sends it to a Content Consumer (i.e., the EHDI registry). The second

Table 2.1 Organizational Roles

Partner Organization	Project Role
CDC	Provide strategic direction and input on project goals and evaluation.
PHII	Provide project management and facilitate project coordination meetings. Collaborate with partners on documentation, evaluation, and dissemination of pilot project outcomes.
OHSU	Implement the IHE EHDI Profile, acting as Device Observation Reporter. Collaborate with project partners on data validation for electronic messages and documents. Provide production EHDI screening data via mutually agreed transport and security mechanisms. Participate in meetings for project coordination and technical implementation. Share information with PHII and OHA on challenges, successes, and recommendations to inform implementations in other jurisdictions and future standards development.
OZ Systems	Implement IHE EHDI Profile, acting as Device Observation Consumer and Content Creator. Collaborate with project partners on data validation for electronic messages and documents. Receive production EHDI screening data via mutually agreed transport and security mechanisms. Generate HPoC documents from screening messages and provide documents to Content Consumer via mutually agreed transport and security mechanisms. Participate in meetings for project coordination and technical implementation. Support project for up to 6 months of production data exchange. Share information with PHII and OHA on challenges, successes, and recommendations to inform implementations in other jurisdictions and future standards development.
OHA	Implement IHE EHDI Profile, acting as Content Consumer. Collaborate with project partners on data validation for electronic messages and documents. Receive production HPoC documents via mutually agreed transport and security mechanisms.

(Continued)

Table 2.1 (Continued) Organizational Roles

Partner Organization	Project Role
	Consume contents of HPoC documents into the EHDI-IS. Participate in meetings for project coordination and technical implementation. Provide a web-based project portal and document repository for the project partners. Share information on challenges, successes, and recommendations to inform implementations in other jurisdictions and future standards development. Collaborate with PHII on the documentation, evaluation, and dissemination of project outcomes.
Lantana Consulting Group	Review screening messages and HPoC documents for conformance to the IHE EHDI Profile and offer consultation to OHA, OHSU, and OZ Systems. Share information with PHII and OHA on challenges, successes, and recommendations to inform implementations in other jurisdictions and future standards development.

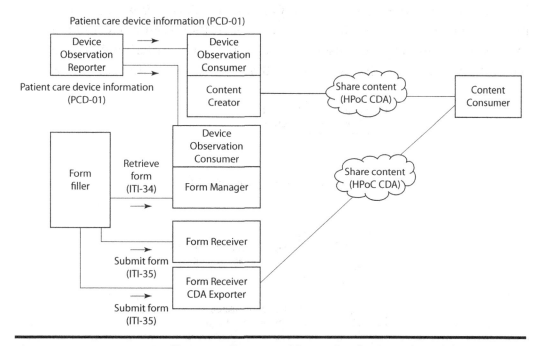

Figure 2.1   IHE EHDI Profile actor diagram with two implementation options. (From http://www.ihe.net/uploadedFiles/Documents/QRPH/IHE_QRPH_Suppl_EHDI.pdf.)

option, RFD, allows for a more manual data entry approach. The form is prepopulated by the EHR if possible, or manually filled in by the EHR user if not, and then sent to a Form Receiver, which then creates the HPoC and forwards it to a Content Consumer.

RFD technology was proposed initially for the Phase 2 pilot as middleware between OHSU and the OHA EHDI-IS, wherein a RFD Form Manager Actor would generate a data capture form within the EHR that is prepopulated with some of the required data. However, the newborn hearing screening results that are already entered into the OHSU EHR newborn assessment flow sheet and into the OVERS birth registry were not available in the EHR standard database, as they needed to be for this project. It was not acceptable to OHSU audiology staff to add a third redundant data entry protocol to their workload, and RFD was another redundant data entry protocol. Further analysis revealed that there was no RFD technology solution available in the EHR production environment. This lead the team to explore alternative approaches.

Instead of RFD, the project partners recommended using PCD-01, the patient care device protocol illustrated in Figure 2.2, which describes the PCD-01 protocol for the Device Observation Reporter for transmitting patient data from devices, such as data generated by hearing screening equipment or other electronic devices, between systems. In this instance, the OHSU EHR assumed the role of the Device Observation Reporter with a human manually entering the data into the EHR, which then communicated that information to the Device Observation Consumer via an HL7 message. So while the Phase 2 pilot followed the pattern described in the PCD-01 option

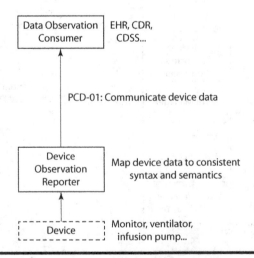

Figure 2.2 PCD-01 protocol. (From http://wiki.ihe.net/index.php?title=PCD_Profile_DEC_Overview.)

of the IHE EHDI Profile, the process did not quite achieve the specification because the data was not sent directly from the hearing screening device.

A project charter developed by the partners helped formalize the initiation of the project and provided definitions of the roles of the partners. Regular status meetings and updates were held and documentation was uploaded to an online forum for collaboration. Participants came together for a site visit in Portland, Oregon, at the end of the project to discuss what they learned and formulate recommendations.

Project Work Plan and Timeline

A work plan was created and maintained throughout the project by OHA. The work plan provided a high-level yet sufficiently detailed list of the necessary steps to complete the project, with tentative targeted and flexible actual deadlines and completion dates. Table 2.2 displays a high-level project timeline for each stage in the project plan.

Table 2.2 High-Level Project Work Plan and Timeline

Stage	Q3 2014	Q4 2014	Q1 2015	Q2 2015	Q3 2015
Process and content evaluation and mapping	X	X	X		
Implement Device Observation Reporter				X	
Implement Device Observation Consumer/ Content Creator				X	
Implement Content Consumer				X	
Develop hearing screening scenarios to assess conformance with standards			X	X	
Validate conformance to standards				X	
Data quality testing				X	
Site visit and lessons learned report				X	X

Privacy and Security Considerations

The Health Insurance Portability and Accountability Act (HIPAA) includes provisions to keep protected health information (PHI) private and secure. This project, like other health information exchange projects, required steps to ensure PHI was handled properly. While OHSU's reporting of hearing screening results to OHA is outside the scope of HIPAA due to OHA's role as Oregon's public health agency, other aspects of information exchange between partners required business associate agreements (BAAs) and virtual private network (VPN) agreements. BAAs allow entities covered by HIPAA (i.e., *covered entities*, typically healthcare providers) to share data with separate entities that are providing some business service. VPN agreements are often required before an organization allows external partners to access secured electronic information.

BAAs and VPN agreements between OHSU and OZ Systems were necessary for handling identifiable patient data, but not between OHSU and OHA because reporting newborn hearing screening results are mandated by statute for all birthing centers with 200 or more births per year. BAAs were not required between OHSU and PHII (who served as project managers) nor Lantana Consulting Group (serving to validate standards conformance), since both PHII and Lantana were covered by the contract between OHA and PHII.

Data Exchange

Clinical Workflow

In order to improve the exchange of data, understanding the context and current workflow that generates newborn hearing screening data is essential.

OHSU is the state's only academic health center, serving more than a quarter of a million patients every year from across the state. OHSU is among the top five hospitals in Oregon for annual birth count, with approximately 2500 infants born every year. OHSU performs hearing screenings on all newborns in their well-baby nursery and neonatal intensive care unit (NICU). The hearing screeners are registered nurses, audiology students, and support staff.

Screeners may use either the otoacoustic emissions (OAEs) test or the automated auditory brainstem response (AABR) test in the well-baby nursery but only the AABR test in the NICU. Screeners affix a label with the results and hand record the results on a multipart paper form, which allows distribution to the family and the infant's primary care provider as well as having other uses. Figure 2.3 displays the first page of the

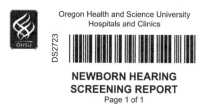

Oregon Health and Science University
Hospitals and Clinics

DS2723

**NEWBORN HEARING
SCREENING REPORT**
Page 1 of 1

ACCOUNT NO.

MED. REC. NO.

NAME

BIRTH DATE

Patient Identification

Dear Parent:

Congratulations on your new baby! As part of your newborn's routine care and as mandated by state law, your infant's hearing was screened using:

❑ Otoacoustic Emissions (OAE)
❑ Automated Auditory Brainstem Response (AABR)

Your Baby:

❑ Passed. No further testing is needed at this time.

❑ Passed, but a follow up hearing screening is recommended in 6 months due to

_____

_____

Your Baby's:

❑ RIGHT ear passed; **LEFT ear needs more testing**

❑ LEFT ear passed; **RIGHT ear needs more testing**

❑ **RIGHT and LEFT ears did not pass and need more testing**

Please call CDRC/Doernbecher Audiology Clinic at 503-418-2116 to schedule an appointment once your child has been discharged from the hospital.

Parent: I have read this information and I understand that I am responsible for scheduling the recommended follow up testing for my baby.

Signature: _____   Date: _____

Screening performed by:

Signature: _____   Date: _____

White-Infant Medical Record   Canary-Mother's Envelope (MBU)   Pink-Audiology Result Folder   Gold-Parent Copy
Canary (DNCC)

03/13 (Supersedes 11/08) Order Number 136901   **DS-2723**

Figure 2.3   OHSU audiology data collection form.

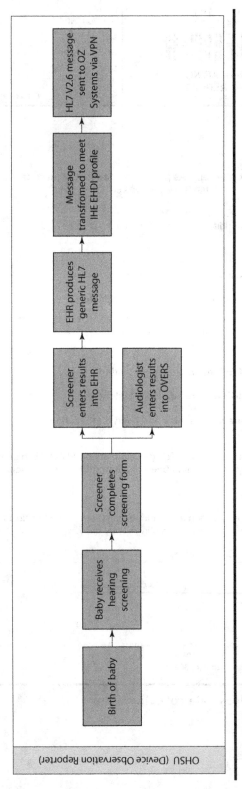

Figure 2.4   Device Observation Reporter screening process task flow.

audiology data collection form used at OHSU. Results are manually entered by the screener into OHSU's EHR. The newborn hearing screening program coordinator at OHSU receives the hardcopy results and enters the information into OVERS.

The current workflow, while allowing for quality assurance in some aspects, also introduces the potential for quality and timeliness challenges, including data entry errors in the EHR and OVERS newborn hearing screening module. This potential for error in either the EHR or the state tracking and reporting database is not unique to OHSU; nor is it likely unique to hearing screening results. Figure 2.4 shows the newborn hearing screening process task flow as the Device Observation Reporter.

EHDI Standard

The IHE EHDI Profile addresses the information exchange needed for an HPoC for a newborn.* The profile specifies the content for an HPoC document. An HPoC records multiple screening tests and the assessment of the screening outcome based on jurisdictionally defined rules. The HPoC provides guidance for future testing or interventions based on the screening results. It also specifies the message constraints for hearing screening devices, such as EHRs, to report screening results.

The HPoC identifies the coding, or vocabulary, standards for data elements, including the specific codes, or value sets, for those data elements. The HPoC persists in its entirety in an unaltered form for as long as jurisdictionally necessary and can be rendered and populated dynamically, as shown in Figure 2.5. HPoC standards are based on CDC reporting requirements and represented by HL7 CDA standards. HL7 CDA is part of HL7's Version 3 family of standards and is not based on HL7 Version 2, which is commonly used by EHRs for messaging. Figure 2.5 describes a partial HPoC and illustrates some of the concepts included in CDA.

To create the HPoC requires that content from the OHA EHDI-IS and OHSU EHR be mapped to the HPoC standard, as demonstrated in the pink column in Figure 2.6, to enable exchanges according to the standard. Similarly, value sets differ across the three entities (OHA, OHSU, and HPoC) and require cross-partner negotiation to reach an agreement on how the codes will be implemented.

---

* http://www.ihe.net/uploadedFiles/Documents/QRPH/IHE_QRPH_Suppl_EHDI.pdf.

Patient	Baby Johnson
Date of birth	July 11, 2014, 04:00:00 –0900
Sex	Female
Race	White
Ethnicity	Hispanic or Latino
Contact info	Primary home: 2345 Desesrt sage road bend, OR 97701 Tel: +1(541)-385-1234
Patient IDs	767767 2.16.840.1.113883.3.969
Document ID	1.3.6.1.4.1.21367.13.20.2144.5142.2165
Document created	July 11, 2014, 16:00:00 –0900
Healthcare service	Hearing screening plan of care at July 11, 2014, 10:26:56 –0900
Author	Thomas clincianson, Mountaineer memorial
Information recipient	45689 2.16.840.1.113883.3.969
Contact info	800 NE Oregon st., Infant hearing program rm. 423 A portland, OR 97232
Document maintained by	OREHDI
Contact info	800 NE oregon st., Infant hearing program rm. 423 A portland, OR 97232

Table of contents

- Hearing screening coded results
- Care plan
- Hearing loss risk indicator
- Problem list
- Procedures and interventions

Hearing screening coded results

Screening date	Screening type	Method	Target site	Result	Reason
7/11/2014 1:20 PM	Neonatal hearing test LEFT (procedure)	OAE	Left ear	Pass	
7/11/2014 1:26 PM	Neonatal hearing test RIGHT (procedure)	OAE	Right ear	Pass	

Figure 2.5   Sample HPoC CDA.

EHDI-IS FIELD	HPoC FIELD	OHSU EPIC FIELD	OHSU EPIC ITEMID	OSHU HL7 FIELD	LOINC CODES	SNOMED CT
LEFT_EAR_RESULT	Result/ interpretation	Hearing screen result-left ear -AABR Test-passed -AABR Test failed -AABR Test referred -AABR Test other -EOAE Test-passed -EOAE Test failed -EOAE Test referred -EOAE Test other	PSD-1000 = FLO:30501356 and FLO:30501368	TBD OBX probably	Left ear (54108-6) -Pass (LA10392-1) -Refer (LA10393-9) -Refused (LA6644-4) -Equipment failure (LA12408-3) -Not performed (LA73044-4) -Not performed medical exclusion-not indicated (LA12409-1)	-Pass (164059009) -Refer (1839244009) -Refused (1839448000) -Equipment failure (1037009008) -Not performed (262008008) -Not performed, medical exclusion-not indicated (410534003)
LEFT_EQUIPMENT_TYPE	Test type	See results OAE or ABR	Hardcoded?	TBD OBX probably	Newborn hearing screening method (54106-0) -Auditory brain stem (response (LA10388-9) -Automated auditory brainstem response (LA10387-1) -Distortion product otoacoustic emission (LA10390-5) -Methodology unknown (LA12406-7) -Otoacoustic emissions (LA10389-7) -Transient otoacoustic emissions (LA10391-3)	

Figure 2.6 Sample data element mapping between EHDI-IS, HPoC, EHR, LOINC, and SNOMED CT.

Table 2.3   High-Level EHDI Data Flow for PCD-01 Protocol

	Capture and Share	*Send*	*Receive, Consume, and Repackage*	*Send*	*Receive and Consume*
Participant	OHSU	VPN	OZ Systems	sFTP	OHA
Role	Device Observation Reporter		Device Observation Consumer/ Content Creator		Content Consumer
Content and Rules	Hearing screening results Demographics Discharge Date		Decision Support Rules		Data Mapping Rules
Input/ Format	Hearing screening results; manually entered		Hearing screening results HL7 V2		HPoC defined by IHE EHDI Profile
Output/ Format	Hearing screening results; HL7 V2.6 Implementation Guide: EHDI Results Release 1		HPoC defined by IHE EHDI Profile		Newborn hearing screening data stored in EHDI-IS

IHE Quality, Research and Public Health Technical Framework Supplement: Early Hearing Detection and Intervention defines how to exchange the data required to populate a newborn's HPoC.* This profile defines document and message content to further constrain the definition of the PCD-01 message.

Pilot Data Flow for EHDI

Table 2.3 provides a high-level description of the data flow across participating organizations using the PCD-01 protocol components of Device Observation Reporter, Device Observation Consumer, Content Creator, and Content Consumer.

---

* http://www.ihe.net/uploadedFiles/Documents/QRPH/IHE_QRPH_Suppl_EHDI.pdf.

```
MSH|^~\&|EPIC|OHSU|RHAPSODY|OHSU|20150526173239-0700|CLAUDERD|ORU^R01|7|T|2.3|||||||
EVN|R01|20150526173239-0700||||CLAUDERD^CLAUDER^DOUG^G^^^^^OHSU^^^^^REGOP
PID|1||E4184^^^^EP-09970897^^^PAO^MR||ROBOTICUS^BABY^^III^^DR.|TRAP^^^|20150428|F|ROBOTICUS^CRUNCHY^ROLL^III|A|123 BABY ST^
PV1|1|I|8NPI^8N20^01^OHSU^D^^^^^|||||||IM|||||||033171^YACKEL^THOMAS^^^^^PAO^^^^DR-1093722928^YACKEL^THOMAS^^^^^^^^^^NP||
OBR|1||||||20150512150000-0700
OBX|1|ST|LA10388-9-L^Hearing Screen Left Ear ABR (Auditory Brainstem Response)^FDC_LN||Not performed, medical exclusion||||
OBX|2|ST|LA10388-9-R^Hearing Screen Right Ear ABR (Auditory Brainstem Response)^FDC_LN||Not performed, medical exclusion|||
```

Figure 2.7   OHSU EHR HL7 message containing newborn hearing screening results (simulated data).

■ Device Observation Reporter: For the IHE EHDI Profile pilot using the OHSU EHR, a newborn hearing screening result HL7 message is generated when data are entered and saved in the EHR. Saving an entry triggers the export of the hearing screening result data to an HL7 message, as shown in Figure 2.7.

The OHSU EHR interface engine transforms the hearing screening result data according to EHDI specifications into an HL7 message, as shown in Figure 2.8. The message is sent via Rhapsody to OZ Systems using a VPN tunnel.

■ Device Observation Consumer/Content Creator: OZ Systems receives and holds all patient result messages until a result message with a discharge flag is received. This occurs when the patient discharge is recorded in the EHR and the resulting HL7 admission, discharge, transfer (ADT) message is transformed into a result message that contains the required discharge flag. Once the message with the discharge flag is received, OZ Systems triggers the creation of the HPoC. The IHE EHDI Profile does not specify a process for triggering the HPoC document. The team selected this methodology based on the tools and capabilities of the participants involved. Figure 2.9 shows an overview of the Content Creator role performed by OZ Systems.

Figure 2.10 shows the coding required to create the HPoC, which is then sent to OHA via Secure File Transfer Protocol (sFTP).

```
MSH|^~\\&|EPIC^1.2.840.1.114350^HL7|OHSU^2.16.840.1.113883.3.2076^HL7|Oz.HL7|OzSystems|20150512155042-0700|C
PID|1||09920001^^^^2.16.840.1.113883.3.2076.2.100||FLOWER^GIRL|||20150512153600|F||2131-1^Other Race^HL70005|
PV1|1|I|12C^12C01^^^OHSU^R||||||NEW|||||||||2038163702\r
OBR|1|09920001201505121500000|09920001201505121500000|54111-0^Newborn Hearing Loss Panel^LN||||||||||||||||||||2
OBR|2|09920001201505121500000|09920001201505121500000|73744-5^Newborn Hearing screen panel of Ear - Left^LN|||
OBX|1|CWE|54108-6^Newborn hearing screen of Ear - left^LN||262008008^Not Performed^SCT||||||D|||201505121500
OBX|2|CWE|73739-5^Newborn hearing screen reason not performed of Ear - left^LN||""||||||D|||20150512150000-0
OBX|3|CWE|54108-6^Newborn hearing screen of Ear - left^LN||164059009^Pass^SCT||||||F|||20150512150000-0700||·
OBR|3|09920001201505121500000|09920001201505121500000|73741-1^Newborn Hearing screen panel of Ear - Right^LN||
OBX|1|CWE|54109-4^Newborn hearing screen of Ear - right^LN||262008008^Not Performed^SCT||||||D|||20150512150
OBX|2|CWE|73742-9^Newborn hearing screen reason not performed of Ear - right^LN||""||||||D|||20150512150000-
OBX|3|CWE|54109-4^Newborn hearing screen of Ear - right^LN||164059009^Pass^SCT||||||F|||20150512150000-0700|
```

Figure 2.8   OHSU IHE EHDI Profile–compliant HL7 message (simulated data).

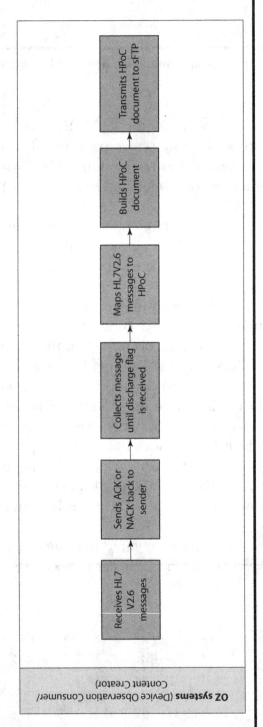

Figure 2.9   Overview of the HPoC Device Observation Consumer/Content Creator process.

```xml
1   <?xml version="1.0" encoding="UTF-8"?>
2   <?xml-stylesheet type="text/xsl" href="CBR.xsl"?>
3   <!-- On Systems - CDA Builder/Exporter v0.986 -->
4   <!-- 2001 NE Green Oaks Blvd, Arlington, TX 76006, United States +1 817-385-0390 -->
5   <!-- Hearing Plan of Care -  cdar2 - 1.1 -->
6
7   <!-- Notes and References relate to both: -->
8   <!-- EHDIOS_14_Specs:Early Hearing Detection and Intervention (EHDI) - Trial Implementation - September 5, 2014 -->
9   <!-- HL7DSTU:HL7 Version 2.6 Implementation Guide Early Hearing Detection and Intervention (EHDI), Release 1 - January 2014 -->
10
11  <?xml-stylesheet type="text/xsl" href="CBR.xsl"?>
12  <?xml-stylesheet type="text/css" href="orcda.css"?>
13
14  <ClinicalDocument xmlns:xsi="http://www.w3.org/2001/XMLSchema-instance" xmlns="urn:hl7-org:v3" xmlns:cda="urn:hl7-org:v3" xmlns:sdtc="u
15    <!-- ***************************************************** CDA Header *****************************************************
16    <realmCode code="US"/>
17    <!-- EHDIOS_14_Specs:Page 44 -->
18    <typeId root="2.16.840.1.113883.1.3" extension="POCD_HD000040"/>
19    <templateId extension="IMPL_CBR2_LEVEL1-2REF_US_I2_2005SEP" root="2.16.840.1.113883.10.20.20"/>
20    <!--<templateId root="1.3.6.1.4.1.19376.1.7.3.1.1.26.1.1"/> HPoC International Realm - urn:ihe:qrph:hpocUV:2013 --><!-- EHDIOS_14_Sp
21    <templateId root="1.3.6.1.4.1.19376.1.7.3.1.1.26.2.1"/> <!-- HPoC US Realm - urn:ihe:qrph:hpocUS:2013 --><!-- EHDIOS_14_Specs:Page 1(
22    <templateId root="1.3.6.1.4.1.19376.1.7.3.1.1.26.2.2.1"/> <!-- HPoC Header Template--><!-- EHDIOS_14_Specs:Page 102 -->
23    <id root="7949360D-89BB-4184-B486-FCC6R09E6BB4"/>
24    <code code="34817-7" codeSystem="2.16.840.1.113883.6.1" codeSystemName="LOINC" displayName="Hearing Screening Evaluation and Managem
25    <title>[HPoC] - Hearing Plan of Care</title>
26    <effectiveTime value="20150204193001"/>
27    <confidentialityCode code="N" codeSystem="2.16.840.1.113883.1.11.16926"/> <!--HL7 BasicConfidentialityKind--> <!-- EHDIOS_14_Specs:P(
28    <languageCode code="en"/> <!-- EHDIOS_14_Specs:Page 44 -->
29    <setId root="7949360D-89BB-4184-B486-FCC6R09E6BB4"/>
30    <versionNumber value="1"/>
31    <recordTarget> <!-- EHDIOS_14_Specs:6.3.2.H1.1 recordTarget - Page 45 -->
32      <patientRole>
33        <id root="1.3.6.1.4.1.21367.13.20.1000" extension="R9879798"/>
34        <addr use="HP">
35          <streetAddressLine>Hearst St. </streetAddressLine>
36          <city>California</city>
37          <state>CA</state>
38          <postalCode>91750</postalCode>
39          <country>US</country>
40        </addr>
```

Figure 2.10 Example of the HPoC document in XML form.

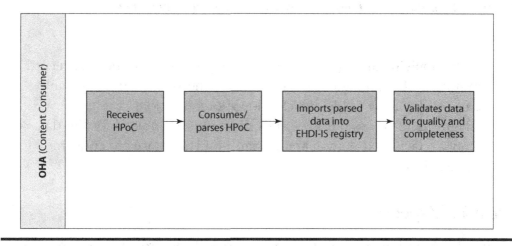

Figure 2.11 Overview of the HPoC Content Consumer process.

■ Content Consumer: Figure 2.11 shows an overview of the HPoC Content Consumer process. OHA receives HPoCs via sFTP. HPoCs are then processed using Model Driven Health Tools (MDHT),* which was developed to promote interoperability standards to extract data and convert contents into a CSV file. The EHDI-IS registry then consumes the CSV

_____
* https://www.projects.openhealthtools.org/sf/projects/mdht.

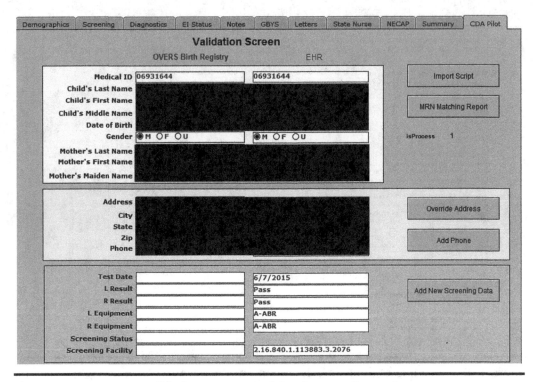

Figure 2.12   EHDI-IS validation screen used for data quality review.

file by applying an algorithm for matching records on medical record number (MRN) and adding data (i.e., hearing screening results) into temporary staging fields, which allows for validation.

Figure 2.12 shows the EHDI-IS validation screen used for the data quality review and demonstrates that the EHR data were consumed into the EHDI-IS.

Technical Aspects

During the planning and development phases of the project, partners developed tools and solutions to aid in sending, receiving, and processing the hearing screening results and the subsequent HPoC. Table 2.4 describes these development tools.

Table 2.4   Development Tools

Organization	Tools	Description/Function
OHSU	EHR	Documents birth and EHDI data elements Triggers result and discharge messages (EHRs can't automatically trigger CDA without a lot of custom work)
	HL7 Mapper/ Validator (Rhapsody)	Maps fields/data elements to HL7 V2.6 specification Transforms HL7 to meet HL7 V2.6 Implementation Guide: EHDI Results Release 1 Validates messages
	HL7 Builder (Rhapsody)	Generates EHDI HL7 message to be sent to recipient
	MDHT	Creates tools to align with EHDI interoperability specifications Extracts the data needed for EHDI processing
OZ Systems	HL7 Emulator	Simulates the creation and receipt of HL7 V2.6 messages Enables testing of the HL7 to HPoC Mapper and HPoC Builder during development
	HL7 to HPoC Mapper	Applies logic Validates message (sends ACK or NACK back to sender) Receives and stores messages
	HPoC Builder	Receives data from HL7 to HPoC Mapper Fills in CDA template Generates HPoC document Validates document against national standards Delivers the document to OHA via sFTP site regardless of validation findings
	Web-based HL7 and HPoC	Permits view-only access to data without the need to download any PHI information Review and validation of the HPoC and corresponding message by SMEs during testing
	sFTP	Sets up and configures a site to transmit HPoC to OHA in a secure fashion

(Continued)

Table 2.4 (Continued) Development Tools

Organization	Tools	Description/Function

OHA	EHDI-IS registry	Development database
		  Maps field/data element
		  Creates new data fields for data collection and
		    import
		  Creates new screens for validation
		  Serves as testing environment
		  Generates reports for processed/unprocessed
		    HPoCs
		  Production database
		  Implements development database changes
		    into production
		  Validates content for quality and completeness

	MDHT	Consumes/parses HPoC Creates CSV file for easy import into EHDI-IS registry
Lantana	HL7 smart tools	Enables user to inspect elements of HL7 message

Evaluation

Standards Conformance Validation

OZ Systems and Lantana Consulting provided support for reviewing and validating screening messages and HPoC documents for conformance to IHE EHDI Profile. The defined set of testing scenarios shown in Table 2.5 was created and used with individual screening result messages. The test scenarios attempted to address frequently occurring real-life scenarios. Each scenario was tested and artifacts were collected and compared to the standards. The findings were documented and contributed to recommendations and lessons learned for the pilot.

Content Validation

Once HPoC data were received by OHA, EHDI staff performed validations to verify the quality and completeness of the HPoC against OVERS. The evaluations included

Table 2.5 Testing Scenarios

Scenario	Artifacts	Tested
0	Preliminary test to validate if testing environment is working as expected.	Yes
A	Expected case: EHR user enters all the hearing data and hits save. The patient is later discharged.	Yes
B	Multiple measurements: The EHR user enters the results over time, perhaps over days. This includes data that have been saved and then edited. The patient is later discharged.	Yes
C	Deleted measurements: Values are entered and saved, but the user then winds up deleting all the values again. The patient is later discharged.	No
D	Discharge without screening results.	No
E	Results without discharge.	No
F	Results after discharge.	No

- A review of the HPoC report generated by OZ Systems
- A comparison of a sample of HPoCs against the CSV file
- An initial evaluation of completeness and correctness using a convenience sample of 20% of the total production data
- A full evaluation of completeness and correctness using the full set of production data received

Results

The EHR interface to capture newborn hearing screening and demographic data for transport to the EHDI-IS was implemented on May 2, 2015, and results capture was activated May 6, 2015.

The first batch of OHSU EHR production data was sent to OZ Systems on June 7 and contained 255 result messages and 251 discharge messages. Of the 506 total messages, 249 HPoCs were produced. The EHDI-IS processed 228 of the 249 HPoCs by MRN matches, resulting in 224 distinct client records due to multiple HPoCs for the same MRN. The Oregon EHDI did not perform a secondary match criteria because of the need to test the validity/quality of MRN matches, and because first-name data in the EHRs were deemed too poor for matching as they almost exclusively contained values such as BOY, GIRL, BOY A, and BOY B.

OHA performed an analysis of the completeness (defined as nonempty fields) and quality (defined as match rate) between the hospital EHR and OVERS data. Specific data elements considered included four demographic fields (Lname, Fname, DOB, Gender), one address field (add 1), and five screening results fields (L result, R result, date, L equipment type, R equipment type).

EHR data were generally more complete than OVERS data, demonstrating the opportunity to improve the timeliness of reporting by receiving data directly from the EHR.

Data quality was assessed by analyzing the match rate for identified fields between EHR data and OVERS. For the purposes of this evaluation, OVERS data were considered the gold standard for two reasons: (1) OVERS contains certified birth data and (2) OVERS hearing screening data are entered by the newborn hearing screening coordinator, who is an audiologist, and thus data undergo a quality review at the time of data entry.

The *DOB* and *gender* fields had very high match rates, at nearly 100%, and 42% of records matched using the *child's last name* field. Only one record matched using the *child's first name* field due to the nearly ubiquitous use of values such as BOY, GIRL, BOY A, and BOY B, as described previously. The low match rate on *child's last name* confirmed our assumptions that (1) *child's last name* can only be used as a secondary match with *DOB* and *gender*, and (2) demographic data from the OVERS birth certificates are better and more complete.

To evaluate the completeness and matching of address data, the *address line 1* field was used. Both OVERS and EHR data fields were 100% complete. However, only 4% of EHR data matched perfectly to OVERS using the initial match criteria of *street number, predirection, street name, postdirection*, and spaces. As a result of the poor match rate using this high standard, a secondary analysis was performed with the match based solely on the *house number* in the *address line 1* field. This comparison yielded a much higher match rate of 92%.

Five data fields were used for the test result analysis: *test date, left result, right result, left equipment*, and *right equipment*. Just over half (52%) of the records matched perfectly on all five test result fields, but almost 40% of the records didn't match any of the fields, indicating probable missing hearing screening data in the hospital EHRs or hearing screening data not yet reported in OVERS. Figure 2.13 displays the completeness and match rate for OVERS compared with the OHSU EHR for each data element.

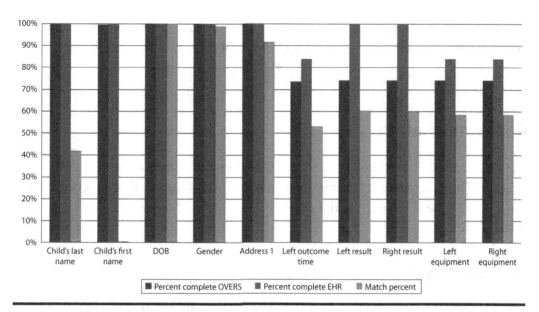

Figure 2.13 Completeness and matching of OVERS and EHR data, selected fields (*N* = 224).

These findings point to some important considerations:

■ Hospital EHR data are not always complete at the time of newborn discharge. Often, parents have not selected a name, which presents difficulties for matching records.

■ MRNs will be heavily relied on for data matching, and their quality and uniqueness will be vital.

■ Data entry errors may occur in hospital EHRs as well as in the public health reporting system. Without a comparison data set, we do not know how extensive these errors may be.

■ Hospitals may be unaware of the degree of data entry errors within their own EHRs and may consider taking steps to assure workflow processes and checks to assure quality data.

■ Workflow and staffing can have a significant impact on data quality and timeliness. It may be necessary to perform a workflow review and implement process changes in order to support a transition from duplicate data entry to relying on hospital EHRs.

■ Using hospital EHRs for public health reporting has the potential to improve the timeliness of reporting.

■ Using hospital EHRs for public health reporting has the potential to reduce duplicate data entry but may be offset by required data audits for ongoing quality assurance.

This analysis suggests that there are a number of considerations that must be taken into account and that transition to interoperability will require more intensive preparation than merely "flipping a switch."

Recommendations

On June 23, 2015, the project team met in Portland, Oregon, to formally debrief. The following recommendations were captured at that meeting and are shared here for future EHDI standards piloting efforts and standards development activities.

Organizational

- Do not underestimate the amount of time required to hire staff and contract with partners after project funding is awarded. The earlier an EHDI program can build partnerships with birthing centers, pediatricians, and audiologists as potential pilot test partners, the better. Also, prior to funding awards, EHDI programs can engage with other programs in their agency to learn how best to hire or partner with health IT subject matter experts that will support the pilot project.
- Because of the sustained and focused attention project staff will need to apply, project funds should be sufficient to support dedicated staff time. Overreliance on "in-kind" contributions from full-time employees will limit the project's impact.
- After an EHDI program has found a willing clinical partner, work with that partner to develop a business case that will help secure participation from the healthcare facility's leadership, IT team, and EHR vendor. That business case should address important goals and priorities. These can include descriptions of how the pilot will lead to reductions in manual data entry time and data errors, improved care coordination and linkages with other clinical settings, and improvements to interoperability infrastructure.
- As the EHDI program works with its clinical partner on a business case, focus on clinical workflow issues that the healthcare facility would like to resolve. As resources allow, also plan on addressing process issues in the public health agency. Ultimately, EHR and public health interoperability standards should be solving real problems experienced by staff members.

■ Look for opportunities to address tasks in parallel. For example, while EHDI subject matter experts identify workflow and data quality issues to solve, IT representatives can resolve security and transport issues for data exchange. Technical concerns related to the movement of data between organizations can, and perhaps should, be independent of the specific content of the data.

■ Another aspect of project management is governance and collaborative decision-making. During the project chartering and kick-off, a process should be developed that will govern how decisions will be reached. This becomes critical at decision points during technical implementation when trade-offs and compromises are necessary. Ideally, the governance process will encourage collaboration and consensus whenever possible. It should also specify a decision-maker when consensus cannot be reached.

■ The project charter and work plan should also specify clear project end points. For example, it could be that the project will be a time-limited trial implementation of data exchange. Alternatively, it could be a longer-term effort to develop ongoing data exchange between production systems. As necessary, the project plan should address how partner engagement will be sustained beyond the milestones outlined in the project plan. Also, there should be consensus on what project outcomes will be evaluated and how.

■ In-person meetings to both kick off and close the project help to build consensus on the project plan, governance, outcomes assessment, and recommendations. Related expenses for these events should be part of the project budget.

■ Limit access to identifiable patient data so that the need for new BAAs between participants is minimized.

Testing

■ The development of test scenarios, including consensus on related workflow issues, may take longer than anticipated. Also, consider the need for multiple rounds of testing and how that will impact the project timeline and budget. The more limited the budget, the fewer test scenarios and rounds of testing, reengineering, and retesting.

■ Consider how de-identified test data for screening results and HPoCs can be retained and reused for benchmark testing, both within a project and through the sharing of artificial data with other jurisdictions.

Reusing test data during the project supports comparisons, as the problems with the pilot implementation are fixed. Sharing test data can help reduce costs and improve preparations for pilots in other agencies.

■ To the extent possible, use actual patient data for the testing scenarios. This will help expose false assumptions about the data and the frequency of scenarios thought to be outliers or "edge cases." At the same time, limit the number of parties that need access to identifiable PHI to reduce the amount of time and effort needed for privacy and security agreements.

■ With respect to projects to pilot test EHDI and EHR interoperability standards, attempt to clarify early what aspects of the standard specifications can be modified for expediency and what aspects are priorities for implementation as specified in the standard.

Standards

The following points are offered as potential change proposals for standards development groups to consider for the IHE EHDI Profile.

■ Make the specifications flexible to accommodate real-time and real-life implementation. This work does not happen in a vacuum. It needs to begin where the EHRs are today and then move toward the complete realization of the standard as EHRs adopt additional data elements that are missing components of the standard, such as risk factors.

■ Send HPoC content via HL7 from EHRs to the state EHDI program. Most EHRs can readily produce HL7 messages and CSV files of EHDI content, but the creation of the HPoC is a challenge for EHR interface engineers.

■ Reposition the creation of the HPoC to the state EHDI program. The state should be responsible for creating the HPoC document and distributing to other healthcare providers as needed and authorized.

■ Establish a testing library that includes a validated de-identified data set for use by other state EHDI programs to test the scenarios against the HPoC.

Conclusion

The EHDI HPoC CDA pilot project demonstrated that a state public health agency could receive and consume HPoCs using real patient hearing screening data generated from a hospital's EHRs and that a pilot project using national standards can be migrated to a production workflow.

The project identified pitfalls in electronic data interchange among multiple partners and the need for coordination among stakeholders from the outset of the project, but also recognized that the project may not be sufficiently prioritized in the clinical space in light of external events, such as an EHR upgrade or key staff jury duty. Even so, the partner organizations in this pilot created and implemented novel tools and solutions for creating and parsing HPoCs, generated new considerations of national guidelines, and identified risks for future implementation.

Having a set of canned test scenarios and data sets for others to use to test an HPoC implementation would streamline the validation process significantly and provide a standard for the evaluation. Know that EHRs may not have the entire set of data elements required by the standard, but it is important to start with the data elements that are available and then work with the clinical partners toward having the EHRs add the missing standards-based data elements to their systems.

A key takeaway for the clinical partner side is that the HPoC creation process is burdensome, impacts a small number of their users, and requires a high level of technical expertise that is not likely to exist at every birthing center. A better path is for the state EHDI programs to accept HL7 or CSV files of data from the hospital EHRs and then create HPoCs at the state level to share as needed and authorized. It is also important to ask if the data need to be real time (as created) or if reporting from the EHRs could occur via the data warehouse the next day. The question is important because it is much easier for the clinical partner staff to pull data from the data warehouse than to create an interface to the live EHRs.

Most importantly, the focus of the initiative should be on data quality rather than transport.

Chapter 3

Renewing Health Project: Telemedicine in the Veneto Region

Claudio Saccavini, Giulia Pellizzon, Mauro Zanardini, and Silvia Mancin

Contents

Introduction

The World Health Organization (WHO), in "Global Status Report on Noncommunicable Diseases 2014" [1], states that the four main types of chronic diseases are cardiovascular diseases (CVDs), cancers, chronic respiratory diseases (e.g., chronic obstructed pulmonary disease [COPD] and asthma), and diabetes. The WHO reported that, as the leading causes of death globally, these diseases were responsible for 38 million (68%) of the world's 56 million deaths in 2012. More than 40% of them (16 million) were premature deaths under 70 years of age. Almost three-quarters of all deaths from noncommunicable diseases (28 million) and the majority of premature deaths (82%) occurred in low- and middle-income countries. During 2011–2025, the cumulative economic losses due to these diseases in low- and middle-income countries have been estimated at $7 trillion. This sum far outweighs the annual $11.2 billion cost of implementing a set of high-impact interventions to reduce the burden of chronic diseases [1].

The global situation highlighted by WHO poses chronic diseases management as a very urgent burden that needs new solutions to be solved. The home monitoring required by the health system to support patient health outcomes and limit resources could be one possible solution.

Many of the most advanced countries in the information and communication technology (ICT) field are trying to find a solution to support the clinical intervention and monitoring of people with chronic diseases. The solutions carried out with the support of ICT are different from country to country, but there are some common characteristics. The devices used could be different depending both on the patient's pathology and on the level of technology chosen. Also, the way to provide the services could be different depending on the actors (GPs, specialists, social workers, emergency departments, or family) that take part in the services.

Although these possible differences exist, most of the services put in place by different countries have the same aim: monitoring the clinical parameters of the patients at home, and moving the patient data to the clinicians with the support of ICT and interoperability. In this way, the clinicians can check the data and make the right decision before the symptoms worsen.

IT Solutions Developed by European Countries

There are a large number of initiatives related to telemedicine all over Europe. It is possible to highlight some differences between European areas—for example, the level of implementation and the care settings involved in the telemedicine systems.

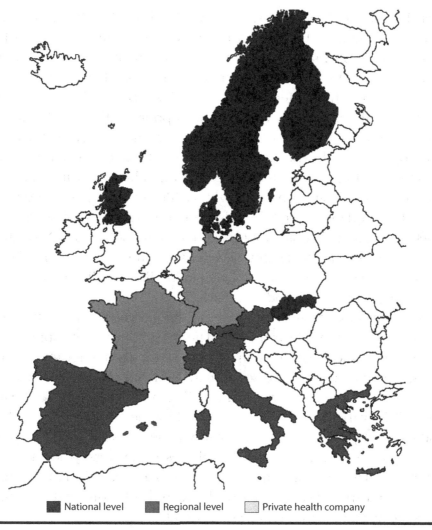

Figure 3.1   Level of implementation in European telemedicine projects.

Considering the level of implementation, a definition of three levels is clear and recognizable in the following map (Figure 3.1).

In Northern Europe, there a prevalence of telemedicine systems implemented at the national level. In Norway, for example, the Norwegian Centre for Integrated Care and Telemedicine (NST) in Tromsø became, in 1993, the national center of competence in telemedicine, which manages telemedicine projects. All the hospitals and GPs are connected to the Norwegian HealthNet (NHN), a secure and dedicated infrastructure for electronic interaction between the health and social sectors. Every day, a patient takes measurements with a portable device. The device then transfers data automatically to a mobile phone for communication to the NHN and is used to register the patient's food habits. If the results show that the glucose level is too low or too high, a clinical alert is sent to the treating physician [2].

In Scotland, NHS 24 [3] is a health board that manages the development of national telehealth and telecare services across Scotland. The Scottish Centre for Telehealth and Telecare (SCTT) [4] is a part of NHS 24, and was established by the Scottish government to support all the health institutions across Scotland; it has supported the implementation of four national telehealth programs (stroke, pediatrics, mental health, and long-term conditions such as COPD). In Scotland, there are also a number of local home monitoring initiatives centering on patients with COPD and congestive heart failure (CHF). All of Scotland's health boards are connected by a single virtual private network called N3 that supports all national applications, providing the security, capacity, and availability necessary for the exchange of information in the health sector. The same implementation line is followed in countries as Finland [5], Sweden [6], and Denmark [7].

If we consider Central Europe instead, the prevalence is related to private health company development. The most relevant examples are Germany and France. For the management of the most relevant chronic diseases, Germany instituted disease management programs (DMPs) on a voluntary basis that were developed by Pflegewerk [8], a German healthcare provider. With variable frequency, indicated by the clinicians, and following individual needs, patients measure vital parameters with devices supplied to them at home, such as wireless blood pressure meters, glucometers, and weight scales. The measures are transmitted to a central health portal, in which GPs and specialists can assess the records of individual patients and where specific alarms are organized and sent.

For France, in 2010, three French private health insurance companies created Vigisanté SAS [9], with the objective of developing telemedicine solutions for managing long-term diseases and reducing health risks. The company proposes screening and healthcare programs combining monitoring from a distance and well-being education, especially concentrated on high blood pressure and other CVDs. The multi-interfaced information system used allows clinicians to manage patient follow-ups using a personalized coaching program, bringing medical information to GPs.

For the south of Europe, countries such as Italy, Spain, Greece, and Austria have chosen telemedicine systems at a regional level. In Spain, thanks to the high level of decentralization, which gives total responsibility for providing healthcare to Spain's 17 regional governments, initiatives related to telemedicine services are taken directly by three main regions;

Catalonia, Basque, and Galicia have been strongly involved in the implementation of telemedicine services for the management of patients with chronic diseases.

The Ministry of Health of the Autonomous Government of Catalonia developed a model of care based on the integration of services and on the definition of care plans for elderly chronic patients, through patient-centered telemedicine services. The Ministry of Health created a single organization (Ticsalut [10]) with the aim to coordinate and act in all telemedicine projects in Catalonia, assisted by a communication network for technological standards. Devices supplied to the patient's home are connected to a mobile phone that works as a gateway to send clinical measurements to the hospital specialist. Individualized programs are managed through a dedicated platform and help ensure adherence to the treatment.

Considering that the Basque population is stratified by taking into account diseases and the level of health service used (the stratification model is similar to Kaiser Permanente's risk stratification model), the specific intervention plans for chronic patients are defined, integrating them into the daily professional's clinical routine.

Osarean, the Basque multichannel health service center, is a project sponsored and managed by the Department of Health and Consumer Affairs of the Basque government; its objective is to increase the number of channels that citizens can use to interact with the health system. This project aims to bring the system closer to the citizens, improving e-health and telemedicine systems in the Basque Country. The services include an ICT platform that allows multichannel interaction with all citizens of the Basque Country and a health system that facilitates all processes, with a focus on the treatment and monitoring of chronic diseases. Several pilots have been successfully implemented for the remote monitoring of chronic disease patients (COPD, asthma, heart failure, and diabetes) and patient empowerment [11].

The healthcare network in Galicia connects all primary and secondary care centers, allowing the use of the same electronic health record (EHR) system by all healthcare professionals, sharing online information such as discharge reports or primary care information. Moreover, the Galician Electronic Health Record System [12] gives all patients access to the information with digital certificates, and in June 2012, the region finished the connection process for joining the national system for EHRs, giving them the capability to interact with other European regions through the European Patient Smart Open Services (epSOS) project (http://www.epsos.eu). The epSOS project, running from July 2008 to June 2014, aimed to design, build, and evaluate a service infrastructure that demonstrated cross-border interoperability between EHR systems in Europe.

There isn't substantial differentiation in the number of settings involved in the telemedicine systems. In Europe, different care settings (primary care, secondary care, and community pharmacies) exist but are not always deeply integrated. The following map describes how the European countries have integrated the settings in relation to telemedicine services and their development (Figure 3.2).

The majority of European countries have telemedicine systems that cover two care settings, in particular the primary and the secondary care. For example, in northern Italy, various initiatives and projects have been developed to create a system for the efficient management of patients with chronic conditions. Investments in the Veneto region were developed to achieve interoperability among telemedicine applications implemented by

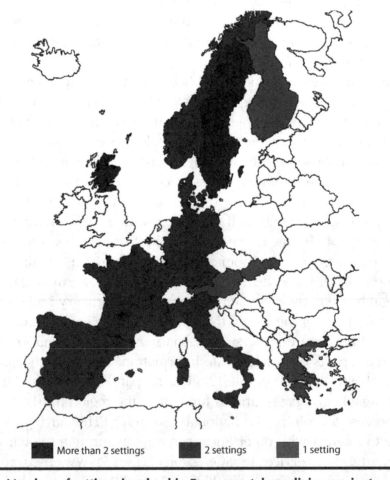

More than 2 settings   2 settings   1 setting

Figure 3.2   Number of settings involved in European telemedicine projects.

the 23 local health authorities (LHAs) and hospital trusts (HTs) [13]. In 2009, an IT integration platform was created through which the 23 LHAs and HTs can exchange patients' documents and images among themselves. It was used for the first time in the context of the HEALTH OPTIMUM project, where the telecounseling service was applied to neurosurgery, telelaboratories, oral anticoagulant therapy, and stroke management [14]. In 2010, the Veneto region began the development of a single platform to monitor patients with chronic diseases.

In southern Italy, telemedicine services are particularly relevant. The Calabria region created two telemedicine initiatives coordinated at the regional level that focused on teleradiology and telecardiology [15]. Territorial and homecare pilot projects have been conducted for the long-term care of chronic conditions and the telesurveillance of frail elderly patients. In collaboration with the National Agency for Regional Health Systems (Age.Na.S.) [16], the Campania and Calabria regions have worked to deliver a comprehensive strategy on telemedicine to support the evolution of the regional healthcare system.

Also, in Denmark, telemedicine services are layered on top of the national electronic health infrastructure. For example, videoconferencing is available on the national electronic health platform to aid hospitals in operation planning between different locations or to support physical cardiac and diabetes examinations for remote islanders. Home care nurses regularly attend to the patient and collect information through a mobile phone. The data are uploaded directly from the mobile phone to an electronic database. The specialist at the hospital examines the received data, then contacts the homecare nurse directly through a secure channel on a computer or phone, and instructs her in the care of each patient [7].

The most advanced system, from the point of view of settings integration, is Sjunet, the Swedish healthcare network, which comprises an infrastructure for communication between hospitals, primary care centers, pharmacies, and homecare. The network guarantees the secure transmission of healthcare data and applications on an IP network separate from the Internet, and it is used for telemedicine, videoconferences, teleradiology, and so on. All hospitals and a large number of primary care centers and pharmacies are connected to Sjunet, which they use for both telemedicine and administrative communication. The patient is supplied with such devices as step meters and those that measure blood pressure, glucose, pulse, and electrocardiogram (ECG), all connected to a tablet PC that the patient can use to check their own measurement trends. The same information is received and displayed by the healthcare staff (clinicians, nurses, GPs) during all the follow-up [6].

With only one setting involved in the telemedicine system, in countries such as Finland [5], the Czech Republic [17], Austria [18], and Greece [19], patients measure vital parameters at regular intervals and send them, through home devices (e.g., mobile phones, blood pressure meters, pedometers, weight scales), directly to the hospital, where clinicians will check the data and plan treatment activities, therapeutic changes, and/or further controls.

RENEWING HEALTH Project

Regions of Europe Working Together for Health (RENEWING HEALTH) was a European project, funded under the Competitiveness and Innovation Framework Programme (CIP)'s ICT Policy Support Programme (PSP), by the European Commission and 20 other partners. Of these 20 partners, 9 are among the most advanced European regions in the implementation of e-health services and in the provision of telemonitoring solutions for chronic patients: Veneto (Italy), Syddanmark (Denmark), the County Council of Norrbotten (Sweden), the Northern Norway Regional Health Authority (Norway), Catalonia (Spain), South Karelia (Finland), the Municipality of Trikala (Greece), the Land of Kärnten (Austria), and the Land of Berlin (Germany).

The objectives addressed by RENEWING HEALTH [20–22] were as follows:

■ Clinical objectives: Improving the quality of life of chronic patients, reducing the need for the patient to use healthcare services
■ User perspective objectives: Providing coherent services that take into proper consideration patients' and professional users' needs, capabilities, risks, and benefits
■ Economic objectives: Containing the cost of care for chronic patients to maintain the sustainability of the health system
■ Organizational objectives: Creating an organizational model for telemedicine services that ensures a safe, clear, and efficient pathway for patients

The aim of the RENEWING HEALTH project was to assess, in real-life settings and with a common rigorous assessment methodology (health technology assessment [HTA] [23]), the use of personal health systems for innovative types of telemedicine services used to monitor chronic patients with CVD, COPD, and diabetes and to prepare them for their wider deployment.

As reported previously, the Veneto region was one of the European regions in which the telemonitoring system was carried out and assessed. In the Veneto region, 20% of the population is over 65 and 10% is over 70, 1.5 million of Veneto citizens suffer from chronic diseases, and 27% of elderly people live alone. These factors increase the use of healthcare resources and the need for social care resources. In the Veneto region, the Social Health Plan act aims to pay more attention to chronicity and to define new models of care characterized by an integration of health and social care. Following this, the Veneto region implemented a unique platform where telecare and telehealth services are integrated. With this platform, the clinical data and social needs of chronic patients are monitored directly from their home.

Veneto Region Telemonitoring Process

The use of telemonitoring allows the remote monitoring of chronic patients directly in their homes, keeping the patient monitored not only for purely clinical aspects linked to the pathology considered. The project provides to healthcare institutions and clinicians a way of offering citizens suffering from chronic diseases more timely and appropriate care wherever they are, and ensures through the permanent monitoring of relevant vital parameters the necessary checks of their conditions to avoid and/or slow down the worsening of their disease and the emergence of complications.

In the Veneto region, a single platform has been developed for the delivery of both telecare and telehealth services (Figure 3.1).

Chronic patients are equipped at home with an emergency button for the real-time detection of emergency situations and with portable devices to measure their clinical data. The portable devices provided to the patients at home are as follows:

■ Wrist Clinic [24]: This is a wireless and all-in-one monitoring system. It measures the heart rate and SpO_2 of patients affected by COPD, and takes blood pressure, pulse oximeter, and one-lead ECG measurements of patients affected by heart failure. This device is applied to the wrist like a wristwatch. Clinical parameters are easily selected, visualized, and displayed. The Wrist Clinic signals correct the working of device both acoustically and visually. When measurements are taken, data are automatically transmitted to the gateway; transmission is wireless, using radio frequencies with a proprietary protocol.

■ Medic Gate gateway: This collects and stores the clinical data from the Wrist Clinic via wireless communication and transfers the data to the regional e-health center via public switched telephone network (PSTN) lines.

■ Digital scale (WS 100): This is used for the measurement of body weight (min. 0.05 kg, max. 150 kg). The weight is automatically measured when the patient steps on the instrument. After each measurement, data are transmitted to the gateway automatically and wirelessly. The transmission happens using radio frequencies with a proprietary protocol.

■ Glucometer (Onetouch® Vita™): This is used as a common glucometer, and the strip is inserted into it by hand. After each measurement, data are available after 5 s in the instrument display with the relative date and time. The glucometer is connected to the gateway by a cable; once connected, blood glucose measurements are automatically sent to the gateway.

■ Alarm device: An emergency device with a red button that the patient can push when needed.

The patient uses the provided devices at home to measure their clinical parameters. The measurements are carried out in accordance with the monitoring plan agreed with the reference clinician at the time of the enrollment of the patient. The monitoring plan shows the days and times in which the patient must perform the measurements. The patients receive two types of training: during the enrollment, the referent clinician explains to the patients and their caregivers the monitoring plan, what type of instruments they will receive, and how use them, then a technician goes to the patient's home to install the gateway and at this time provides the second level of training. The technician tests all the devices with the patient and explains again how they work.

Relating to Figure 3.3, the telemonitoring service is provided through the following steps:

■ Step 1–2: The patient takes measurements with the provided clinical devices following the plan agreed with his or her clinician. The telemonitoring devices collect data and send them to the gateway device.

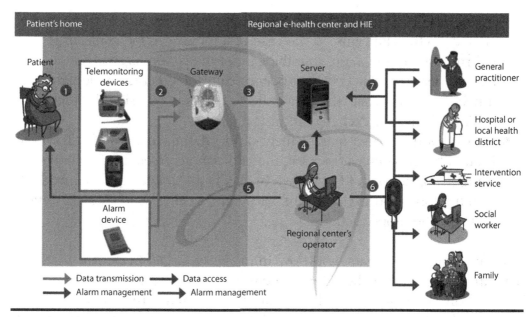

Figure 3.3 Telecare and telehealth platform.

■ Step 3: The gateway device transmits data collected by the patient to the server of the regional e-health center, where a group of operators are in charge of data management.

■ Step 4: To handle the data received, the operators refer to the monitoring plan defined by the reference clinician. The monitoring plan is shared with the e-health center at the moment of the enrollment of the patient. In this way, the operators know when the patients have to take the measurements, what type of measurements they have to take, and the alarm thresholds. They verify whether the patients have taken the expected measurements and if any alarms have occurred. The center's operator checks the data sent by the patient, accessing them through the homecare portal. In cases where the clinical parameters are out of normal range, the telemonitoring software detects the alarm situation and the operator manages it following the standard protocol.

■ Step 5: In alarm situations, the operator contacts the patient to verify the alarm and assess the situation.

■ Step 6: If the alarm is verified, and depending on its severity, the operator can forward the alarm to the GP, the specialist, and the social worker. The alarms are managed following the rules of triage. In the case of a green alarm, where the parameters are slightly out of the normal range, the clinician receives an email that warns of a variation.

In the case of a yellow alarm, in addition to the email, a telephone call is made to the clinicians. In the case of a red alarm, the clinician is informed about the alarm, but the care of the patient is switched to the telecare services. The center's operator calls the emergency department if needed. In any case, the data collected are shared using the regional health information exchange infrastructure.

◼ Step 7: For the proper management of the alarm situation, after the notification by the center's operator, the clinician accesses the data collected using his or her own EHR system, which is integrated with the regional health information exchange infrastructure, to check the patient's data and take the proper actions.

Clinical data as well as workflow information are collected in a structured way so that the reference clinician can find the following information: the date of the alarm, alarm value, alarm threshold, action taken by the doctor, the date of the closure of the intervention, the trend of the measurement for the patient, changes in the monitoring plan, pending referrals, and so forth. The clinicians can access those data at any time, allowing him or her to effectively monitor the patient's health conditions.

Relating to Figure 3.1, the telecare service is provided through the following steps:

◼ Step 1: In case of emergency (social or health), the patient pushes the emergency button to trigger an alarm.
◼ Step 2: The alarm device sends the alarm signal to the gateway.
◼ Step 3: The gateway device transmits the alarm to the regional e-health center.
◼ Step 4: The center's operator checks the alarms sent by the patient, accessing them through the homecare portal.
◼ Step 5: The operator manages the alarm situation, contacting the patient to verify the alarm. If the alarm is verified and depending on the severity or nature (social and/or clinical aspects) of the case, the operator contacts the patient's family and the emergency and/or social service department.

The center's operators also call the patients periodically to monitor their life conditions and quality of life.

From a Research Study to a Healthcare Service

The RENEWING HEALTH project was a clinical research study that involved about 7000 chronic patients enrolled in the nine European countries described previously. The Veneto region involved more than 3000 patients. All these patients were followed for 12 months by cardiologists, pulmonologists, diabetologists, nurses, GPs, and social workers. As explained previously, the aim of the RENEWING HEALTH project was to assess the services provided following the HTA guidelines [23].

The results obtained from the Veneto region have proven that for chronic patients with a specific clinical condition, monitoring their clinical data improves their status and decreases the number of hospitalizations and specialist visits. These results also imply an economic saving for both the healthcare system and the patient.

During the study phase, the perception of the clinicians was also assessed. This evaluation pointed out three main issues that should be addressed using ICT methods:

■ Clinicians need to dynamically share monitoring data between all the clinical actors involved in the care of the patients.
■ Specialists need to consult telemonitoring data directly from the hospital's electronic medical record (EMR).
■ Clinicians should be able to affect the evolution of the monitoring process—for example, asking for referrals.

These needs arose after the study phase and implied the development of another type of integration between the systems involved: a workflow management infrastructure.

Workflow Management Infrastructure

When the sharing of clinical data is not enough to grant system interoperability, there is a need for a standardized platform to share workflow information. A workflow management system provides an infrastructure for the setup, performance, and monitoring of a defined sequence of tasks, arranged as a workflow. In the e-health world, this means that systems involved in a clinical workflow are able to understand the state of progress of a specific task and can contribute to the workflow following predefined rules. Usually a workflow within an organization does not need to be supported by a standardized platform because it relies on site-defined rules and is affected by organizational aspects that reduce the value added by IT standards.

This scenario is quite different in a cross-enterprise environment, in which systems that belong to different organizations want to share workflow information with other participants without exporting the complexity of the local workflow, only providing the minimal set of data useful to the progress of the workflow itself.

Integrating the Healthcare Enterprise (IHE), a healthcare IT standards development organization, has identified a specific integration profile that is able to address these needs: Cross-Enterprise Document Workflow (XDW) [25].

IHE Approach to Clinical Workflow Management: XDW Profile

The XDW Profile enables participants in a multiorganizational environment to manage and track the tasks related to patient-centric workflows as the systems hosting workflow management applications coordinate their activities for the health professionals and patients they support. XDW builds on the sharing of health documents provided by other IHE Profiles such as Cross-Enterprise Document Sharing (XDS), adding the means to associate documents conveying clinical facts to a patient-specific workflow. XDW provides a common interoperability infrastructure that supports a wide range of specific workflow definitions. It is designed to support the complexity of health service delivery with the flexibility to adapt as workflows evolve. This profile defines an instrument called a *workflow document* to manage and track a shared workflow. It records the creation of tasks and maintains a historical record of tasks as they move through the associated workflow. The workflow document also maintains the references to health information input and output associated with each task. Such shared workflow status information allows the various participating systems to coordinate their actions by

- Being aware of the history of a workflow for a patient
- Obtaining and reading the workflow's incomplete tasks
- Updating this shared document as the workflow tasks are performed according to a referenced workflow definition

XDW offers a common, workflow-independent interoperability infrastructure that

- Benefits many clinical and nonclinical domains by avoiding different competing approaches to workflow management
- Provides a platform on which a wide range of specific workflows can be defined with minimal specification and application implementation efforts on the workflow definition (e.g., medical referrals workflow, prescriptions workflow, homecare workflow)
- Facilitates the integration of multiorganizational workflows with the variety of existing workflow management systems used within the participating organizations
- Increases the consistency of workflow interoperability and enables the development of interoperable workflow management applications where workflow-specific customization is minimized
- Offers the necessary flexibility to support a large variety of different healthcare workflows by not being overly constrained

In accordance with this, the XDW Profile is a suitable tool to create a workflow management infrastructure focused on the *care pathway* of the patient. The care pathway can be considered an XDW because it involves many participants belonging to different organizations. The telemonitoring process is just one step in the healthcare story of the patient, and it develops as a workflow conditioned and triggered by other processes such as prescriptions, referrals, data acquisitions, and so on.

As it was defined by IHE, the XDW Profile requires another layer of standardization to be really effective and applicable to a real scenario: a common workflow definition shared between workflow participants.

XDW Documents as Tools to Manage/Orchestrate a Clinical Workflow

The structure of a workflow document is organized into *tasks* and *task events*.

A task describes an activity, or a group of activities, that need to be accomplished or have been accomplished. A task is characterized by several attributes:

- The type of task
- The owner of the task
- The current status of this task (one of the status values that are valid for this task)

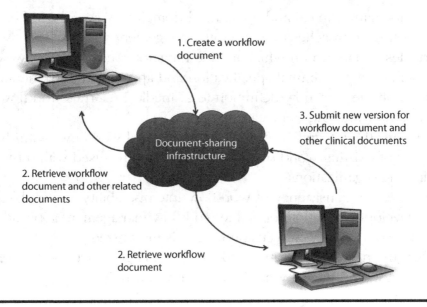

Figure 3.4   IHE XDW workflow management approach.

- The references to documents used for input or produced as output
- The history of past task events for this task that document the progress of the task up to the present state

When a person or organization has been assigned as the owner of a task, the task is placed under execution (Figure 3.4). When the expected activity/activities is/are completed successfully, the task status is changed accordingly. A task event is a record of a change (of status and/or other attribute) of a task; a task event history is the list of task events for a specific task.

As shown in Figure 3.5, the XDW document is structured into two parts:

1. General workflow information about the document
2. Tasks that are completed or not yet completed in the workflow, as well as, for each task, the related task events that track its progress

Task and task event specification leverages a proper subset of the task model and specification from OASIS Human Task, a standard closely related to well-known workflow standards such as BPEL (http://docs.oasis-open.org/bpel4people) and BPMN (www.bpmn.org).

The task and task events include references to clinical or administrative input and output documents to the task or task event.

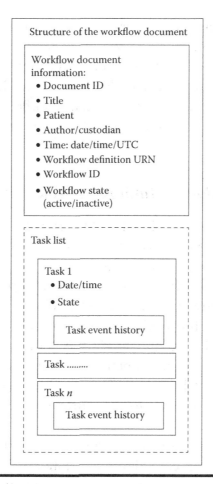

Figure 3.5 Workflow document structure.

■ The *input* attribute contains references to documents that are relevant for workflow participants in performing the task. For example, for a performed examination, this could contain a reference to a referral request. It may also contain references to *parent* workflows to which this workflow is a *child*.

■ The *output* attribute contains references to documents that were produced as a result of performing this task. For example, this could contain a reference to a report written by a specialist. It may also contain references to child workflows initiated by this workflow as a parent.

At any time, if a participant chooses to update the workflow for a specific patient, it shall either create one or more new tasks or update an existing task and record a past task event. Each update to the workflow document results in a new instance of the workflow document, which is published as a replacement of the previous version. The prior version being replaced is then placed in the status *deprecated* so that only the newest workflow document is active. When a new workflow document is created, the Content Creator assigns it a workflow identifier. This workflow identifier does not change during the evolution of the workflow itself, and allows the grouping of all the XDW documents that belong to the same instance of the workflow.

Standardized Workflow Definition for Telemonitoring Processes

During the development of the RENEWING HEALTH project, and due to results obtained by the pilot, it was decided to identify a suitable way to transform the telemonitoring platform into a shared services suite accessible to all patients. Many different organizational approaches related to the telemonitoring process were analyzed by collecting input from the IHE international community involved in the patient care coordination (PCC) domain. This collaboration culminated in the drafting of a new workflow definition profile called the Cross-Enterprise TeleHome Monitoring Workflow Definition (XTHM-WD) [26].

The objective of this profile is to standardize

- Workflow participants: Any system/person that can be involved in the workflow and that can condition its evolution
- Workflow tasks: Each task (human or applicative) that needs to be accomplished to complete the workflow
- Workflow-allowed evolutions: Each available transition between tasks

All the systems that are involved in the telemonitoring workflow agreed on the whole set of rules defined in the workflow definition profile. Figure 3.6 describes the full process flow defined in the XTHM-WD Profile.

The standardized process flow is created by four main phases:

1. Service activation: This phase involves a request for the activation of a telemonitoring service and the subsequent approval.
2. Telemonitoring management: In this phase, monitoring data are collected and reported.
3. Alert management: If an alert is detected, this condition should be managed by a doctor of reference that can take four decisions: no action, a

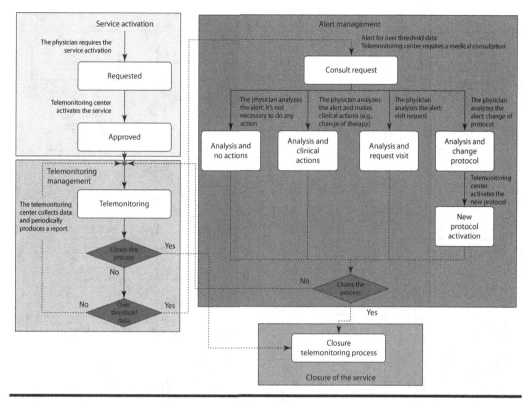

Figure 3.6   Telemonitoring process flow.

non-predetermined clinical action, request a referral, change the telemonitoring protocol.
4. Closure of telemonitoring process: This task is performed when the
patient does not need the service anymore.

Each event of the process is tracked in a related update of the workflow
document. Figure 3.7 describes workflow document updates during the
routine telemonitoring process, which involves the request for a telemonitoring *service activation* (Step A), the approval of the service activation (Step B),
and the multiple collections of telemonitoring data (Step C1).

Veneto Region Telemonitoring Platform

The telemonitoring platform built in the Veneto region is based on a *publish and subscribe* infrastructure provided by the regional health information exchange (HIE) system. In software architecture, *publish and subscribe*
is a messaging pattern where senders of messages, called *publishers*, send

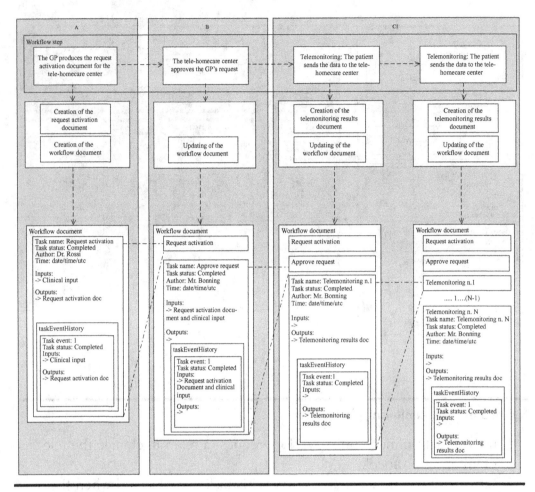

Figure 3.7   Workflow document updates.

messages directly to specific receivers, called *subscribers*, but publish messages to other systems, without knowledge of which subscribers, if any, there may be. Similarly, subscribers express interest in some resources and only receive messages that are of interest, without knowledge of which publishers, if any, there are. The document-sharing infrastructure of the Veneto region is based on an XDS.b environment that allows the sharing of clinical documents produced by 23 LHAs. This standard has been chosen as the more common and diffused solution to sharing documents among many different hospitals.

Using the same approach, the identified telemonitoring participants (GP's EHRs, hospital EMRs, social workers, and homecare operators) can access the telemonitoring workflow related to a specific patient. Each system involved is able to consume the content of the telemonitoring workflow

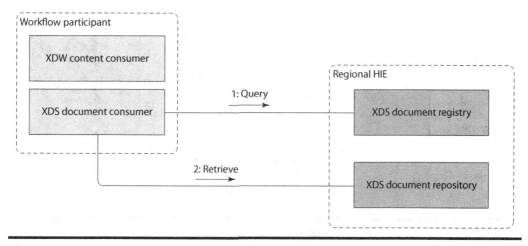

Figure 3.8 Query and retrieve process flow.

document, viewing the entire history of the patient related to the telemonitoring service (Figure 3.8).

If the system is identified among the active participants of the workflow, it can also affect the evolution of the workflow itself. An actor can contribute to the workflow, updating it and submitting the updated version to the document-sharing infrastructure (Figure 3.9).

Every new publication of workflow-related documents triggers the creation of notifications that are sent to all the participants involved in the workflow itself (Figure 3.10).

This process is based on the interoperable infrastructure defined by the Document Metadata Subscription (DSUB) Profile [27]. Monitoring data are stored in a document that is structured in accordance with Health Level

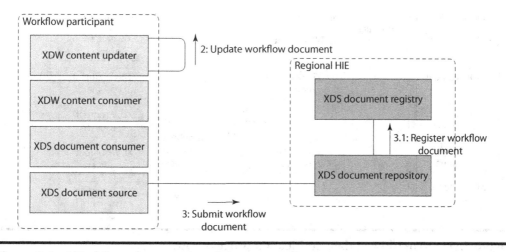

Figure 3.9 Workflow document update process flow.

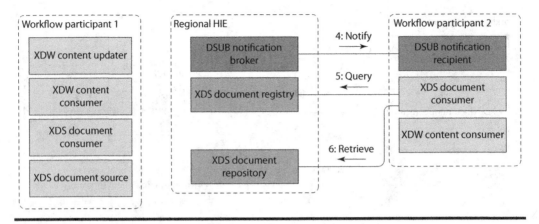

Figure 3.10   Workflow creation notification process flow.

Seven International (HL7)'s "Implementation Guideline: Personal Health Monitoring Report" (PHMR) [28] (Figure 3.11).

Workflow information and monitoring data are automatically acquired by systems involved in the telemonitoring process.

Use Case Scenario Description

A patient that meets inclusion requirements is identified as a potential user for the telemonitoring service by the GP of reference. In this case, the GP will use his or her EHR system to create a new workflow document that tracks the status of the telemonitoring process (request for activation pending) as well other clinical documents useful for evaluating the request of

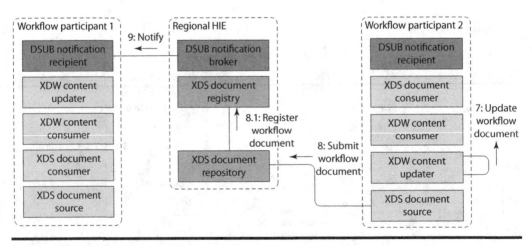

Figure 3.11   Workflow update notification process flow.

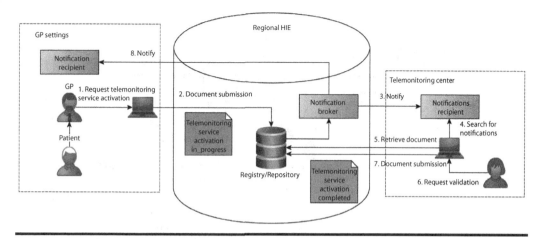

Figure 3.12   Activation of telemonitoring service data flow.

activation of the telemonitoring service. The regional telemonitoring center is notified and evaluates the request (consuming the request document and related clinical documentation).

If the *activation* is approved (in accordance with regional policies), the workflow document related to the telemonitoring process is updated accordingly. The GP is notified of the activation so that he or she can proceed with the enrolling steps (Figure 3.12).

When personal devices are installed in the patient's home, he or she can begin the acquisition of data. Data are sent using a gateway to the telemonitoring center, where they are stored and validated (this can be done by an operator or by a software system). Each acquisition involves the creation of a PHMR by the telemonitoring center, and the workflow document is updated to track it. Each participant in the workflow (the GP and eventually a specialist) is notified of each acquisition and has the possibility to monitor the health status of the patient (Figure 3.13).

If a critical condition is detected by the telemonitoring center, a request for a consultation is created, asking for a clinical action made by the GP. The GP is notified of the consultation request so that he or she can refer to the collected data and take the proper clinical action (e.g., change the monitoring protocol) (Figure 3.14).

The telemonitoring center is notified of the update to the monitoring protocol and an operator can apply an appropriate action to fulfill the GP's request (e.g., change the acquisition timing, change the threshold, etc.).

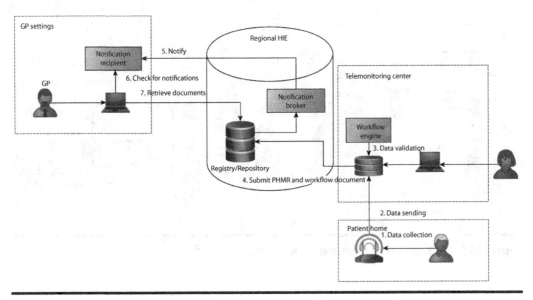

Figure 3.13   Telemonitoring data collection and validation data flow.

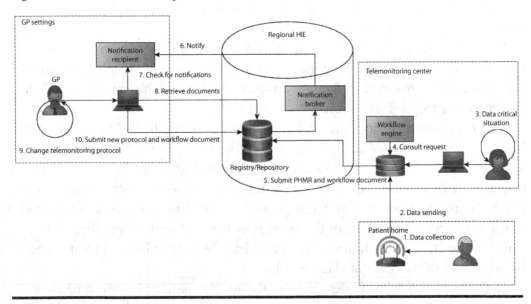

Figure 3.14   Telemonitoring protocol update data flow.

Conclusions

The main goal of the RENEWING HEALTH project was to assess telemonitoring services based on ICT technologies under various aspects. All the trials showed that the interventions used were at least as good as the usual care from the clinical point of view and provided considerable enhancement in the effective interaction between clinicians and patients. There are positive trends in the improvement of what causes hospitalizations, rehospitalizations, specialist visits for pathology, and instrumental examinations for the group of patients treated with telemedicine. For patients affected by CHF, the quality of life measured with the SF36 questionnaire is improved in the group treated with new services [29]. The telemonitoring infrastructure allowed clinicians to be engaged in the process when needed. Devices utilized by the patients were generally well received by participants; hence the services were not regarded as a replacement for usual care but were considered added value. Professional users have demonstrated great advantages in having a shared and interoperable platform to manage clinical and workflow data.

- Clinicians didn't perceive the new functionalities as an additional load on daily activities because data are integrated directly into their EHR system.
- Clinicians are promptly notified of adverse situations.
- Having a clear and standardized approach to manage the workflow reduced the time needed to resolve adverse situations.

Home care services and the enhancement of the patient's role in his or her treatment are the most interesting areas in which European healthcare IT projects are working. The HIE project in the Veneto region is evolving in order to cover, with the same infrastructure built for the RENEWING HEALTH project, additional clinical pathways such as the monitoring of sports/physical activities and chronic diseases.

References

1. WHO, Global status report on noncommunicable diseases, http://apps.who.int/iris/bitstream/10665/148114/1/9789241564854_eng.pdf, p. xi.
2. http://www.telemed.no.
3. http://www.nhs24.com.
4. http://sctt.org.uk.
5. http://www.eksote.fi/eng/Sivut/default.aspx.
6. http://www.swedish.org.
7. http://www.southdenmark.com.
8. http://www.pflegewerk.com.
9. http://www.vigisante.com/index.aspx.

10. http://www.ticsalut.cat/en_index.
11. http://www.osakidetza.euskadi.eus/r85-ghhome00/es.
12. http://www.sergas.es.
13. http://www.regione.veneto.it.
14. http://www.consorzioarsenal.it.
15. http://www.regione.calabria.it.
16. http://www.agenas.it.
17. http://ntmc.cz/?CTRL=about.
18. http://www.kabeg.at.
19. http://www.e-trikala.gr/en.
20. http://www.renewinghealth.eu.
21. Mancin S, Saccavini C, Dario C, Centis G. Telemedicine for the remote monitoring of patients with chronic disease: European project RENEWING HEALTH. *Int J CARS* (2011) 6 (Suppl 1): S305–S366.
22. Mancin S, Centis G. Integration of telehealth and telecare: The implementation model for chronic disease management in the Veneto region. *Studies in Health Technology and Informatics* (2014) 200: 56–61.
23. http://www.renewinghealth.eu/assessment-method.
24. http://en.medic4all.it/our-services/modular-services/check-up-and-prevention.
25. http://ihe.net/uploadedFiles/Documents/ITI/IHE_ITI_Suppl_XDW.pdf.
26. http://ihe.net/uploadedFiles/Documents/PCC/IHE_PCC_Suppl_XTHM-WD.pdf.
27. http://ihe.net/uploadedFiles/Documents/ITI/IHE_ITI_Suppl_DSUB.pdf.
28. Implementation Guide for CDA Release 2.0 PHMR.
29. Dario C, Luisotto E, Dal Pozzo E, Mancin S, Aletras V, Newman S, et al. Assessment of patients' perception of telemedicine services using the service user technology acceptability questionnaire. *International Journal of Integrated Care* (2016) 16(2): 13. DOI: http://doi.org/10.5334/ijic.2219.

Chapter 4

Immunizations

Alean Kirnak

Contents

Introduction

Immunization standards provide an excellent opportunity to look at what happens when different stakeholder groups develop different standards for a shared healthcare domain in which they must ultimately cooperate. This is the case in the 25-plus-year history of immunization standards. Immunization registry architects, developers, managers, and users pioneered a set of messaging standards to use in exchanging data with provider source systems, on which public health data is dependent. As they evolved, electronic health record (EHR) companies evolved their own methods of sharing a broad spectrum of healthcare data with each other, based on their largely private sector requirements. The US Meaningful Use incentive program accelerated both types of exchange—those of providers with each other and those between providers and public health—raising the still-unresolved question of how those standards will work seamlessly with each other. Even before that challenge is resolved, standards development efforts arising from other requirements in other environments complicate the topic even further.

The task of explaining not one but a set of immunization standards—multiple versions of Health Level Seven International (HL7) standards, Integrating the Healthcare Enterprise (IHE) profiles, Service-Oriented Architecture (SOA) standards, and the emerging Fast Healthcare Interoperability Resources (FHIR)—in itself is a challenge. In the end, the HL7 Service-Aware Interoperability Framework (SAIF) provided some broad guidance by dividing interoperability issues into *dimensions**:

---

* HL7, "HL7 Service-Aware Interoperability Framework: Canonical Definition Specification, Release 2," DSTU, May 2012. http://www.hl7.org/documentcenter/public_temp_49D16A77-1C23-BA17-0C9D9903321EB07E/standards/dstu/SAIF_CANON_DSTU_R2_2012MAY.pdf.

1. *Enterprise*: For instance, stakeholder group requirements
2. *Information*: For example, demographic and immunization data
3. *Behavioral*: What function systems on each side of the exchange are expected to perform
4. *Engineering*: Including deployment examples
5. *Technology*: What specific standards are implementable in which environments

The rest of this chapter will move through the various immunization standards roughly in chronological order of their development, touching on the preceding five topics. One of the most subtle dimensions—behavioral—turns out to be the most useful in exploring the similarities and differences among immunization standards. This chapter describes all the standards in terms of the primary behaviors required by all users of immunization information, and highlights how some newer standards support behaviors not required by earlier ones. Successful interoperability, not only among systems implementing a common immunization standard but also among groups of systems who have evolved different shared standards, depends on bridging that gap in behavior.

Immunization Registries

Today's immunization standards began with immunization registries. An *immunization registry* is a central repository of original or copies of immunization records generated by healthcare providers of a common geographic, jurisdictional, or organizational area. Examples of coverage areas include a country, state, or county; a private provider such as Kaiser Permanente; or the US military. Immunization registries emerged in the United States in the 1990s. A term that is used within the immunization registry community, but which has never caught on outside it, is *immunization information system* (IIS). Because of its wider use, *immunization registry* will be used here.

Immunization registries were created by public health entities to help control vaccine-preventable diseases. Unlike many population or hospital registries, immunization registries were intended to provide recommendations in real time at the point of care. The motivation is to help providers improve coverage rates in the population with the eventual goal of reducing disease outbreaks. For this, providers need access to

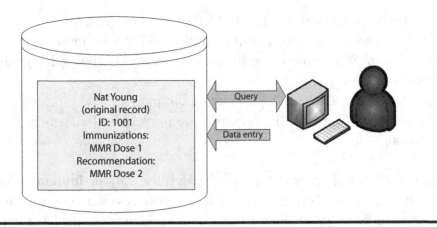

Figure 4.1   Early immunization registries.

patient immunization records, both their own and those given by other providers. An immunization registry was conceived as a central data repository of patient immunization records shared among providers in a community.

When immunization registries appeared in the mid-1990s, the primary means of capturing data was through user data entry screens (Figure 4.1). This presented a challenge to adoption since the point-of-care users on whom data entry relied were located at provider sites where vaccines were given. The "low-hanging fruit" therefore tended to be public health clinics and safety net providers that were under the control of the same organization that housed the registry and whose users could access the screens via the public health local area network. To make screens available to remote providers, private telecommunication (T1) lines were sometimes extended; in other cases, data was entered remotely into a desktop application and periodically synchronized. Faxed immunization records that were entered after the fact by immunization registry staff provided a method of last resort.

Bidirectional communication between emerging EHR systems and immunization registries was at first a futuristic and long-term goal that became the driving requirement for immunization interoperability standards.

Business Requirements

The classic business requirements for immunizations are found in the "Record Immunization History" storyboard of the "HL7 Version 3 Domain

Analysis Model: Immunization, Release 1" (the Immunization DAM).* Well-written and well-vetted, it is quoted here:

> Susan Q Public has moved from Portland, Maine to Augusta, Georgia. She brings her son to his new pediatrician on 1/1/2011. The clinic staff enters his demographic information into the office EHR and requests an immunization history from the State IIS. No record is found. Susan has a paper record from the previous pediatrician. The record includes the following:
>
> Date of birth: Feb 2, 2009

Vaccine Group	1	2	3	4	5
HepB	2/2/2009	4/2/2009	8/3/2009		
DTAP	4/2/2009	8/3/2009			
Polio	4/2/2009	8/3/2009			
HIB	4/2/2009	8/3/2009			
Rotavirus					
MMR	2/1/2010				

> Clinic staff enters this information into the EHR and transmits it to the State IIS. They request an evaluation of this history based on the ACIP schedule and request a forecast of what doses are due next from the State IIS. The State IIS returns an evaluated history and forecast of next doses due. They determine that they will administer a Pentacel (DTAP/HIB/IPV) dose, Lot number Q234sw in the right deltoid intramuscularly. The manufacturer is Sanofi Aventis. This administration is recorded in the EHR system. The EHR system transmits this to the IIS. The IIS incorporates this new information into its data store.

This storyboard illustrates the target usage of immunization standards in an interoperability environment and touches on the data and primary functions that they must support.

---

* http://www.hl7.org/documentcenter/private/standards_temp_82A3DCFE-1C23-BA17-0CA445A2D3289D8E/v3/V3DAM_IZ_R1_INFORM_2012MAY.pdf.

Data Elements

Immunization data includes those required to support the business requirements, broadly including

- Patient identifiers
- Demographic information, such as name and date of birth of the patient as well as of relatives and responsible parties
- Immunization data, including the patient's immunization history, as well an evaluated immunization history, a recommendation for next vaccines, and contraindications and precautions
- Header or wrapper information, such as the identification of the sender and receiver, message dates and identifiers, and so forth

Behavior

Certain broad capabilities are common to most or all immunization registries, including *data exchange, record matching and consolidation*, and *decision support*, described as follows.

Data Exchange

Immunization standards must support bidirectional data exchange as follows:

- The submission of immunization records
- The retrieval of consolidated patient histories and next vaccines due at the point of care

The preceding storyboard contains specific references to the contemporary ideal of data entry into an EHR and data exchange with the immunization registry. It includes both queries and updates, as depicted in Figure 4.2.

Query: The clinic staff enters his demographic information into the office EHR and requests an immunization history from the State IIS. No record is found.

Update: Clinic staff enters this information into the EHR and transmits it to the State IIS.

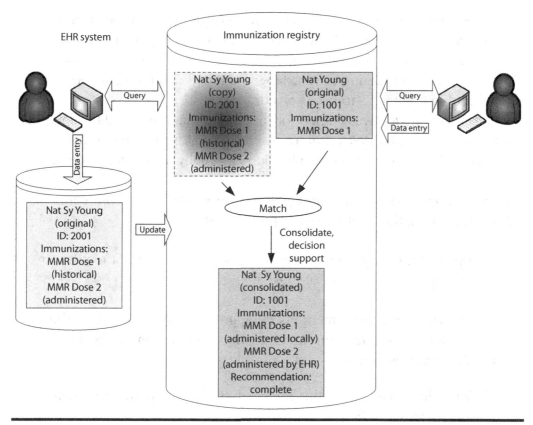

Figure 4.2   Immunization registries and EHRs.

Matching and Consolidation

Recall we defined an immunization registry as storing both original and copies of immunization records. This is conceptually similar to an original paper document versus a copy. Let's consider the original records to be those of the type generated through the early user screens shown in Figure 4.2. In such a situation, the immunization registry records the only original electronic copy of a patient's record. By contrast, the records entered into an EHR and transmitted to the immunization registry constitute copies, since the originals are stored on the EHR system.

One can imagine early data entry screens that allow users to enter, retrieve, and edit a patient's record—say, for the patient Nat Young. This is like a "living document" that is updated by different people from time to time. All the users, regardless of their organizational affiliation, access Nat Young's single immunization registry record.

Once copies of records entered elsewhere begin to arrive by electronic interface, a challenge arises. Now, a record for Nat Young arrives on an interface, *and* a record for Nat Young already exists in the registry. Do they refer to the same Nat Young or not? How are those two records—one an original and one a copy—to be resolved?

The term *duplicates* was coined for the notion that this plurality of records is superfluous and *de-duplication* for the process of turning them into a single, consolidated record. De-duplication is actually a two-step process:

1. Determining that records belong to a common patient, or *matching*
2. Consolidating them into a single patient history

In the preceding storyboard, matching is suggested, but not explicit, in both the query and the update of these text excerpts:

> *Query*: The clinic staff enters his demographic information into the office EHR and requests an immunization history from the State IIS. No record is found.

> *Update*: Clinic staff enters this information into the EHR and transmits it to the State IIS.

The choice of the term *duplicates* in itself suggests that all but one of the records for a single patient is redundant. This first notion is indicated in Figure 4.2 by the fact that the consolidated record retains the original immunization registry ID of 1001. The EHR record copy, with ID 2001 as assigned by the EHR, "disappears" into the consolidated (1001) record. It is implementation-dependent whether any or all of the EHR (2001) record is permanently retained. Figure 4.2 suggests that the EHR ID of 2001 is in fact retained, so that when changes to the record arrive from the EHR, they may be correctly associated with the immunization registry record identified as 1001.

A subtle, contrasting notion is that each of the records in the plurality is equally important and valid, and none is actually redundant. This second notion is depicted in Figure 4.3. Note that the consolidated record is derived from the two source records, 1001 and 2001, and assign a new identifier, 3001, which is associated with the individual person Nat Young.

This distinction will become important later in this chapter when standards behavior evolves to the point of linking matched records instead of merging them. Figure 4.2 depicts the basis for a merged approach; Figure 4.3

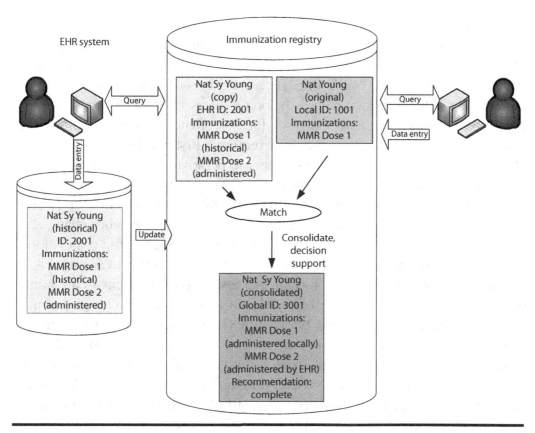

Figure 4.3 A second approach to de-duplication.

depicts a link. In the meantime, from the user's point of view, the consolidated records of Figures 4.2 and 4.3 appear the same either way.

Matching

Immunization registries and other systems use *matching algorithms* to decide whether two records belong to a common patient. Matching algorithms are heuristics; that is, the matches they make are correct most of the time, but they can be wrong, just as a fingerprint match or even a DNA match can sometimes be wrong.* Matching algorithms typically rely on demographic data—for example, name, date of birth, address—but as we shall see, they can leverage any useful information, including identifiers, visit dates, and other data. For this reason, the data elements used in matching are sometimes referred to as *traits*. Generally speaking, the more detailed and accurate the traits, the better the match.

---

* Identical twins have the same DNA, and there are very small possibilities of other errors.

Matching algorithms strive to compensate for the fact that traits tend to be entered and stored a little differently by different organizations. Note that the EHR user enters Nat Young's name as "Nat Sy Young," while the immunization registry user enters it as "Nat Young." The matching software models a judgment call as to whether two records belong to the same person or not. For example, one implementation may look for exact matches on the first, middle, and last names, while another may only require a first and last name match. Matching algorithms vary from deployment to deployment in the data elements they consider and in how much discrepancy they tolerate in matched values. They are constantly being tuned. Matching algorithms can change over time as new data sets are added or as the tolerance for mismatches changes.

Matching algorithms are sensitive to the demographics of the population to which they are applied. They may be tuned, for example, to accommodate ethnic variations on name format. Names of Spanish origin—common in southern California—include both the mother's and father's names, sometimes resulting in several strings being stuffed into a data entry field that was designed for a single first, middle, or last name. Distinguishing individuals of multiple births—twins, triplets, and so forth—is another common challenge in pediatric systems.* The demographic data of such children may almost entirely align: same parents, dates of birth, addresses, visit dates, and only a slight variation in first names that could just as easily be a misspelling. More will be said about twin matching in the section on IHE Pediatric Demographics.

Assigning a unique identifier to each person, such as a social security number (SSN), does not necessarily solve the problem. In countries where a national patient identifier is well established and consistently used, the need for complicated matching algorithms is reduced but seldom eliminated. The caveat is due to domain, privacy, and data quality issues. For example, in Canada, identifiers are assigned on a province-by-province rather than a national basis. In Australia, the individual healthcare identifier (IHI) is widespread in billing records but just beginning in clinical records. In the United States, SSNs are subject to widespread falsification, duplication, privacy issues, and inconsistent inclusion in the electronic medical record. And then, of course, there are simple data entry errors.

Matching is implied any time a new patient record arrives at the immunization registry, and possibly again when it is updated. Matching is also implied when searching a registry for existing records.

---

* Just as it can be a challenge separating identical twins using DNA.

Consolidation into a Single Patient Record

Once a group of records is identified as belonging to a common patient, they need to be consolidated to provide a logical and complete view of that person's immunization history and a recommendation as to the next vaccine the patient should receive.

The ways of choosing which demographic fields to include in the consolidated records are as diverse as the matching algorithms. The most recent data may be given priority, or the most complete, or the most frequently appearing across the set of records. Consolidating immunization histories is a bit different. Providers tend to record not only the immunizations they give but also those the patient has received elsewhere in the past. The former are called *administered* records, the latter *historical*. Consolidating immunization records is often a question of giving priority to the administered records and suppressing the historical ones. Historical and administered records are true duplicates.

Note the demographic data and the administered and historical vaccines of Figures 4.2 and 4.3. The immunization registry user gives Dose 1 of MMR to Nat Young and records it (administered). The EHR user makes a note of MMR Dose 1 (historical), then gives MMR Dose 2 and records it (administered). In creating the consolidated immunization history, the immunization registry software ignores the historical and displays the two administered records. "Nat Sy Young" is chosen over "Nat Young" in consolidating the demographic information. Why? It's up to the developers of the software to decide which data value to keep and which to discard, based on some criteria. Perhaps it's because "Sy" provides a middle name and is judged to be more complete, or perhaps it's because "Nat Sy Young" arrived later and is considered more up to date.

Decision Support

Finally, immunization registries have from inception included a decision support feature, although the term *decision support* was not used in the early days by the immunization registry community. *Decision support* is now a general term applied to intelligent or knowledge-based systems in healthcare and other applications, but in the 1990s, immunization registries used the terms *algorithm* or *vaccine forecast module* (VFM) when talking about the software that recommended, or *forecasted*, the next vaccine. Such software encodes an interpretation of clinical guidelines for administering immunizations. The acronym VFM is still used in the immunization registry community, even though within provider circles, *forecast* can be used in reference to vaccine or other healthcare product inventory. *Recommendation* or *care plan* is the more common private sector terminology to describe a future course of patient care action. The VFM assists in scheduling the next provider appointments, issuing reminders, and evaluating patient status as up to date or not.

The VFM is a complex but potentially high-value service of the immunization registry because it quickly answers the questions caregivers most frequently ask:

■ What vaccines are due now?
■ When does the patient need to come back for the next one?

These questions are not always so simple to answer. The vaccine best practices, published by physician groups and guided by the Centers for Disease Control (CDC), are open to substantial interpretation. Decision support systems by contrast are *state machines* that need unequivocal, or *deterministic*, transitions among a finite set of states. They expect a specific recommendation to be defined for every possible combination of facts about the patient that could come into play: demographics, vaccine history, contraindications and precautions, and so forth. It is doubtful whether all possible such combinations have ever been enumerated in the guidelines, let alone tested and documented; the mathematics of the possible combinations suggests that there may be too many of them.

In other words, immunization decision support services are, like matching algorithms, essentially heuristics, and are subject to the same variations, constant tuning, and need for human oversight that matching is. For this reason, most immunization registries have historically retained a staff physician who uses his or her judgment to describe rules and define VFM test suites with their desired outcomes. These rules are then transformed into a computable format and verified against the test cases. Standardized test suites, developed by a collaboration of clinicians, have only recently begun to appear.* Standardization of the VFM is still a bit ahead of the state of the art.

The decision support feature can be seen in the following storyboard:

> *Decision support*: They request an evaluation of this history based on the ACIP schedule and request a forecast of what doses are due next from the State IIS. The State IIS returns an evaluated history and forecast of next doses due.

---

* CDC, "Clinical Decision Support for Immunization (CDSi)," November 15, 2016. http://www.cdc.gov/vaccines/programs/iis/cdsi.html.

Decision support is responsible for generating the next vaccine recommendations illustrated in the preceding drawings.

The HL7 2.3.1 Guide

Background

In the early days of immunization registries, gaining the much-desired participation of private providers was challenging. Some of the obstacles included the following:

1. Legal: Immunization registry participation was encouraged, but not legally required, in most regions. In addition, state laws impose differing privacy and other requirements in different states.
2. Economic: The expense to providers of *double data entry* and connectivity was high. Widespread commercial availability of the Internet around the turn of the century helped but didn't necessarily eliminate the cost of recording their own records and entering data into the immunization registry as well. Revenue sources that justified the cost were hard to identify.
3. Clinical: Although there was general agreement that electronic records had at least the potential to provide better data, the traditional *yellow card* or paper copy was often good enough. Until adoption attained critical mass, it may have even been superior; sparsely populated immunization registries provided incomplete histories. In any event, little harm was perceived in readministering vaccines for which the patient had no verifiable record.
4. Technological: The uptake of EHR systems was slow. The pioneers tended to be the larger providers, more prevalent in the United States on the west coast. Even when EHR systems were available, provider IT resources were competitive. Immunization registry interface projects suffered when ranked against more critical clinical needs with better financial return.

Data exchange standards were seen as one way to increase the repeatability of EHR–immunization registry interfaces and reduce cost.

The Legacy of Susan Abernathy

The earliest immunization standard to achieve wide success was the "Implementation Guide for Immunization Data Transactions Using Version

2.3.1 of the Health Level Seven (HL7) Standard Protocol."* Susan Abernathy is named therein as the CDC contact and is recognized as the driver for its development. We will use the shorthand *2.3.1 Guide* henceforth to avoid having to repeatedly spell out its lengthy title.

Early versions of the 2.3.1 Guide were maintained by a loosely organized group of immunization registry professionals called the Committee on Immunization Registry Standards and Electronic Transactions (CIRSET), which operated informally.† The role of implementation guides was less well defined within HL7 than it is now; as such, the 2.3.1 Guide was used by agreement among the CIRSET members and with the support of the CDC, but it was not a balloted standard of any American National Standards Institute (ANSI)-accredited organization.

Prior to the publication of Version 2.2 of the 2.3.1 Guide‡ in 2006, CIRSET was absorbed into the American Immunization Registry Association (AIRA). At the urging of several CIRSET members, AIRA joined HL7 and began sending representatives to working group meetings. This provided AIRA with more context as to what was being done in HL7 generally, as well as access to other HL7 members and resources.

2.3.1 Guide Message Set

In keeping with the technology of the times, support for the three major behaviors—data exchange, matching/consolidation, and decision support—are entirely contained within the two primary messages of the 2.3.1 Guide:

1. Unsolicited Vaccine Record Update (VXU)
2. Query for Vaccination Records (VXQ)

Figure 4.4 refines Figure 4.2 to show how the EHR system uses the VXQ and VXU messages to implement our storyboard and fulfill our business requirements. Note that the immunization registry user does *not* use VXQ and VXU to query and update the records. The use of messages in this

---

* "Implementation Guide Version 2.0" is dated June 1999: http://www.ihs.gov/RPMS/PackageDocs/ GIS/hl7guide610.pdf.
† CIRSET is described in *Public Health Informatics and Information Systems* by Patrick W. O'Carroll et al. as "an association of immunization registry developers who are actively developing data exchange capability with other registries and providers and have agreed to follow the HL7 implementation guide" (New York: Springer, 2003, p. 480).
‡ Not to be confused with Version 2.2 of HL7.

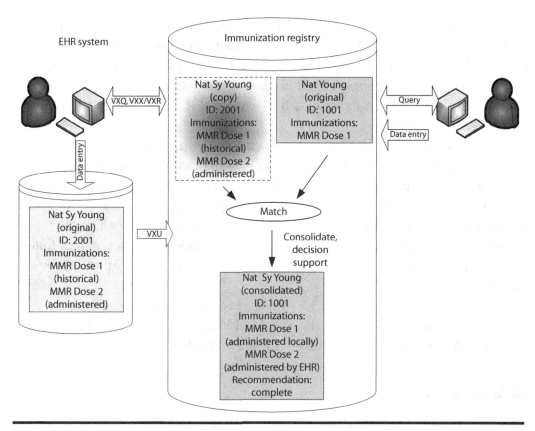

Figure 4.4 VXQ and VXU.

discussion implies the existence of two separate systems. The immunization registry users of Figure 4.2 are connected directly to the system that stores the records and so have no need for messaging.

An HL7 Version 2.3.1 VXQ sends search criteria to the receiving system in order to retrieve an immunization record. The criteria may include a patient identifier, demographic data, or both. The receiver uses matching software to find the record(s) that best fit the search criteria and returns them to the sender. The results of a VFM on the retrieved record may, optionally, also be returned.

When a patient identifier is included in the VXQ search criteria, the receiving system returns either nothing or a single matching record, since identifiers are presumed to identify a unique patient. When only demographic search criteria are provided, a set of possible, or candidate, matches may be retrieved. HL7 2.3.1 provides for two types of return messages, a VXX and a VXR. The 2.3.1 Guide specifies that a VXX message be returned when two or more possible matches are found, and a VXR when a single match is retrieved.* The intent of VXX is to allow the user to choose the correct patient from a pick list then query again, this time sending the identifier of the selected record. An identifier match, or a high-confidence demographic match, is sometimes called an *exact match*. Since the second VXQ contains an identifier, an exact match is expected to be found and returned in a VXR.

An HL7 Version 2.3.1 VXU message sends an immunization record, including patient identifier, demographic information, and immunization data, to the receiving system. It is implied, but not stated, that the receiving system will use the identifier(s) and the demographic data elements to match the transmitted record to a current record, if any, and merge or link the transmitted one with the retrieved one.† Is also implied, but not stated, that the newly recorded record is then available for use by the VFM and to be returned in future queries.

There is no particular HL7 2.3.1 message whose sole purpose is to request the results of the VFM; the vaccine forecast may optionally be returned in the VXR along with the immunization history.

Behavioral Analysis

The 2.3.1 Guide support for the three major immunization registry behaviors we have identified is summarized in Table 4.1.

As a way of understanding the significance of specifying behavior in standards, consider the subtle implications of the specified use of VXX versus VXR return messages. Recall that on receiving a VXQ, the 2.3.1 Guide instructs the receiving system to return a VXX if two or more candidate matches are retrieved, and a VXR if only one is found. The intent of this model is unspecified in the standard. It might have been chosen to minimize the number of trips between the requesting and responding system. Whatever the intent, a common inference is that if only one match is found, it is an exact match.

Note the subtle logical error in this interpretation. When the search is done on demographic data, as opposed to an identifier search, a single match could be an exact match or a potential match.

---

* If no matches are found, only an acknowledgment is returned.
† Note that VXU includes a message header segment that, under HL7 Version 2.3.1, includes both merge and link/unlink trigger events. Hence, either the merge or link is theoretically supported.

Table 4.1   2.3.1 Guide Behavioral Analysis

Data Exchange	
Query	VXQ
Update	VXU

Match and Consolidate
The standard is silent, but the receiving system is assumed to perform matching in response to both a VXQ and a VXU.

Decision Support
The standard supports no specific message whose sole purpose it is to invoke the VFM, but the output of the VFM may optionally be returned in a VXR when a single matching record is found in response to a VXQ.

Suppose for a moment that the "Nat Young's" of Figure 4.4 are actually two different people, as illustrated in Figure 4.5. A VXQ query might specify "Nat Young" as the search criteria, resulting in the retrieval of two potential matches, returned in a VXX. The user will see two possible choices, choose one based on the correct date of birth, then issue another VXQ query and retrieve the immunization history detail for the correct patient.

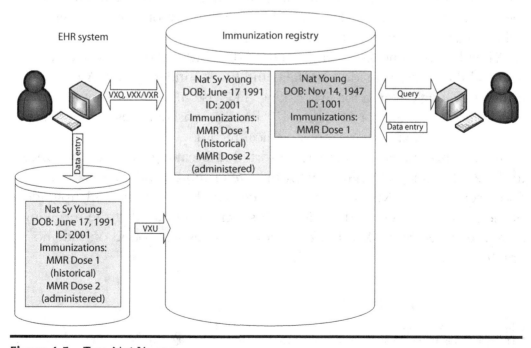

Figure 4.5   Two Nat Young.

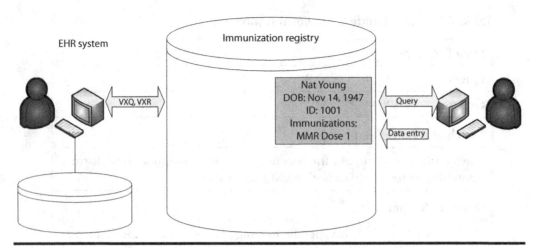

Figure 4.6   Returning VXR when only one record is found.

Imagine, however, that the VXQ query is issued by the EHR user prior to creating the initial record for Nat Sy Young born in 1991, as illustrated in Figure 4.6. The record for Nat Young born in 1947 is a potential match to the search criteria "Nat Young," even if the user is really looking for Nat Sy Young born in 1991. Without specifying the date of birth in the search criteria, the software can't tell. This time, since there is only one potential match, the immunization history is immediately returned in a VXR. This can lead the user to mistakenly conclude that the returned, complete record signals a definite match, when in fact it has not.

When he finally notices that the returned record is the wrong one, he may feel the software made a mistake and lose confidence in it. A user performing a Google search for "Nat Young" likewise may or may not initially realize the software error of Figure 4.7,* but the consequences are more serious when misled about a patient's medical record.

To sort this out, some registries resorted to breaking their conformance to the 2.3.1 Guide, returning a VXX on *one* or more candidate matches and reserving the VXR for an exact match. The HL7 Version 2.5.1 upgrade of the 2.3.1 Guide resolved the issue. It specifies instead that the receiving system is to return a VXX if *one* or more matches was found on a demographic query.

---

* The Nat Young in the photos was in fact named after the Nat Young described in the text. Both are famous competition surfers, just of different generations.

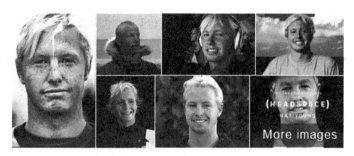

Nat Young

Author

Robert Harold "Nat" Young is an Australian surfer and author. Born in Sydney, New South Wales, Young grew up in the small coastal suburb of Collaroy. Wikipedia

Born: November 14, 1947 (age 68), Sydney, Australia

Spouse: Ti Young

Movies: Crystal Voyager, Palm Beach, Endless Summer Revisited, More

Children: Beau Young, Bryce Young, Nava Young, Naomi Williams

Figure 4.7   Which is the correct Nat Young?

IHE Profiles

Background

By 2007, electronic interfaces between private provider EHR systems and public health systems were still the exception rather than the rule. In an effort to remove the barriers to such connections, the Public Health Data Standards Consortium (PHDSC), which operated out of Johns Hopkins University, initiated a collaboration with IHE. IHE was organized by EHR and IT infrastructure companies to find the least common denominator by which healthcare systems could communicate with each other "out of the box." IHE denies that it develops standards; instead, it builds *profiles* for specific use cases, utilizing existing standards when available. The IHE Technical Framework specifies the IHE Profiles and the *transactions* they use. Profiles constrain standards to remove ambiguity and emphasize the most important elements. PHDSC, with a group of collaborators, initiated the development of profiles for interfacing with public health.

Although public health and private providers share common interests, the requirements of the IHE stakeholder group differ somewhat from those of public health organizations. Just as the 2.3.1 Guide was influenced by public health requirements and immunization registry design, the IHE Technical Framework reflects the requirements and approaches of its private sector stakeholders. Where population health tends to be divided along the lines of its initiatives—immunizations, epidemiology, chronic disease, and so on— private providers must focus on the individual patient. They must therefore have a total picture of the patient's health at the point of care.* Public health looks for broad results over a population and so may be more concerned with obtaining voluminous data, even if there is some minor inaccuracy within it, whereas professional and liability concerns require private providers to emphasize accuracy in records of individuals and to clearly isolate data they are responsible for from those of another provider, even when records are shared.

Unlike HL7, which allows projects to take whatever time they need, IHE follows a strict annual cycle. Committees vote on profile proposals at the beginning of each year. IHE Profiles define the business requirements they are meant to solve and specify the necessary solution. The goal with regard to immunizations was to be able to support use cases such as that described in the previous storyboard. Unsurprisingly, the first immunization profiles pitched by the PHDSC collaborators supported the primary immunization registry behaviors we have identified.

- Data exchange
- Matching and consolidation
- Decision support

Among these are an Immunization Content (IC) profile, and a Pediatric Demographics enhancement to the Patient Identifier Cross-Referencing (PIX) and Patient Demographic Query (PDQ), and a decision support profile called Request for Clinical Guidance (RCG).

IC defines the format for immunization-specific data exchanges within an IHE infrastructure profile called Cross-Enterprise Document Sharing (XDS). XDS shows up over and over again in IHE deployments and is the basis for data exchange across a broad spectrum of clinical domains. PIX and PDQ are also core profiles that address the required matching and consolidation functionality. RCG was a new profile that was deferred by the public health team to the second IHE planning year.

---

* Some immunization registries also track related public health information such as body mass index (BMI), tuberculosis testing, and so forth.

IHE Technical Framework

The IC, XDS, PIX, PDQ, and RCG profiles are collectively part of the IHE Technical Framework. The IHE Technical Framework reflects concepts and advances not in common use when the 2.3.1 Guide emerged 10–15 years earlier. The technological shift is substantial in at least three major areas: the separation of concerns, the concept of documents versus messages, and the concept of record merging versus linking. The deployment example of Figure 4.8 illustrates this shift.

Separation of Concerns

Separation of concerns has to do with breaking functionality into small units that are reused in a variety of combinations to satisfy business needs. We saw that in the 2.3.1 Guide, both of the primary messages, VXU and VXQ,

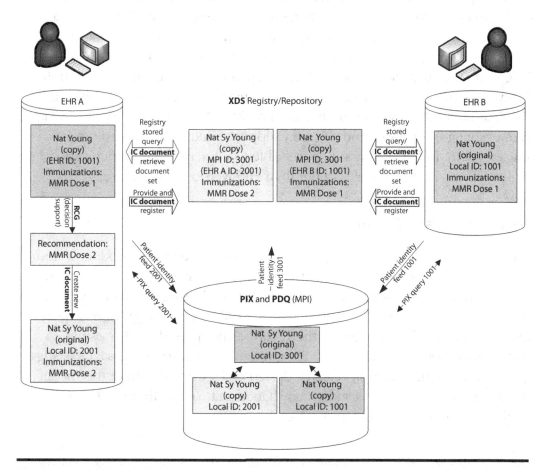

Figure 4.8   IHE technical framework immunization standards example deployment.

trigger all of the major behaviors of immunization registries—data exchange, record matching and consolidation, and decision support. By contrast, the IHE Technical Framework provides separate profiles for different behaviors. More complex behavior is built from more granular transactions. These building-block transactions create economy through reuse and allow deployments to be configured in a variety of ways in different situations.

Separation of concerns is a foundation for the highly successful technical approach known as SOA. An IHE white paper* entitled "A Service-Oriented Architecture (SOA) View of the IHE Profiles" illustrates the parallels between the IHE Technical Framework and SOA. It relates the IHE Technical Framework to SOA principles and to the SOA standards described later in this chapter.

In Figure 4.8, the three primary behaviors of immunization registries—data exchange, matching and consolidation, and decision support—that were in our previous deployment examples carried out by a single immunization registry are now performed by three different systems. This might make sense in an environment in which, for example, record matching is carried out for a variety of purposes by a common subsystem. As an example of reuse, note that the Patient Identity Feed (ITI-8) transaction is accepted both by the PIX Cross-Reference Manager and by the XDS Registry/Repository. As an example of flexibility, note that the immunization decision support functionality is initiated by the EHR rather than by an immunization registry. Yet in another deployment, data exchange, matching, and decision support could all be carried out on a single system. In fact, it is not inconceivable to implement an immunization registry based on IHE profiles rather than HL7 Version 2 messaging.

Messages versus Documents

The IHE profiles leverage a highly successful HL7 Version 3 product called Clinical Document Architecture (CDA). CDA meets many of the aforementioned requirements of private providers. Where messages are ephemeral, documents are persistent. A message exists only long enough to transport information, which is parsed by the receiver, interpreted, and possibly transformed before being stored. The ephemeral nature of messages is suggested in the immunization registry design of Figure 4.2, where the incoming Nat Sy Young record is shown as shaded out, suggesting most of it isn't retained after processing (Figure 4.9).

---

* http://www.ihe.net/Technical_Framework/upload/IHE_ITI_TF_WhitePaper_A-Service-Oriented-Architecture_SOA_2009-09-28.pdf.

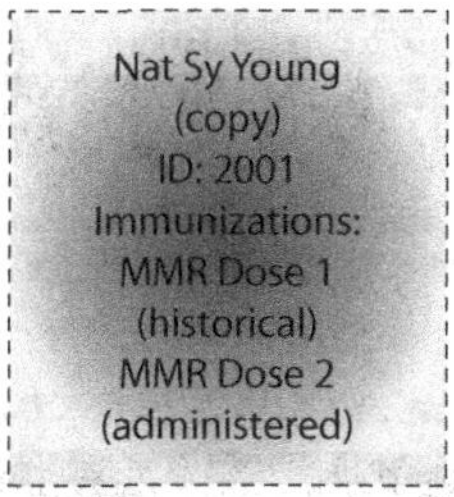

```
Nat Sy Young
(copy)
ID: 2001
Immunizations:
MMR Dose 1
(historical)
MMR Dose 2
(administered)
```

Figure 4.9 The message containing Nat Sy Young's record is not preserved after processing.

A document, by contrast, is designed to be stored in its entirety just as it is, associated with a particular person or organization entrusted with their maintenance.

Documents are human readable, so they do not need to be parsed in order to be displayed. Figures 4.10 and 4.11 illustrate the human-readable and partial source renditions of an IC document, respectively. The human-readable version is the way it would be displayed in a browser; the source is what you might see if you clicked on the "view source" option in your browser. The CDA structure supports a wide palette of healthcare information, including lab results, procedures, medications, and others, as well as immunizations.

Because of their properties of *persistence, wholeness, stewardship,* and *potential for authentication,** documents enforce the fidelity between the original and copies of immunization records. Let's state that again: *the copies of the documents created and sent by the EHR are preserved in their entirety within the shared XDS repository, until the source EHR—and only the source EHR—decides to update them and send replacements.* In this sense, the behavior of document-based solutions is more like the immunization registry design of Figure 4.3. In fact, note that the XDS Registry/Repository of Figure 4.8 contains *only* copies of immunization records and, unlike both Figures 4.2 and 4.3, does not support any direct editing of the documents it manages.[†]

Merging versus Linking

A final major technological advance embodied by IHE profiles over the 2.3.1 Guide lies in their explicit support for record linking. The two options

---

* Gay Giannone, "Introduction to the Clinical Document Architecture," Alschuler and Associates, June 2009. https://www.hl7.org/documentcenter/public_temp_AE357077-1C23-BA17-0CA75E4B05D80954/wg/pedsdata/Alschuler_CCD_May09.ppt.

[†] Technically, the XDS Registry/Repository does "edit" document *metadata*, just not the documents themselves.

SEBASTIAN DOS SANTOS - HISTORY OF IMMUNIZATIONS for DOS SANTOS, SEBASTIAN

Document Information

Detail:

Title:	HISTORY OF IMMUNIZATIONS for DOS SANTOS, SEBASTIAN
Description:	HISTORY OF IMMUNIZATIONS *(11369-6)*
Effective Date:	Thursday, August 25, 2016 at 6:42 :20 am

Patient Information

Patient Detail

Name:	SEBASTIAN DOS SANTOS	**Patient Number:**	10082522
Address:	123 Encanto	**Date of Birth:**	Thursday, August 16, 1990 at 12:00 :00 am
	San Diego , CA 92021	**Gender:**	Male
	United States		
Home :	(619)111-2222		

Immunizations

Name	CVX Code	Date Admin	Dose #	Mfg Code	Lot Number	Route	Site
		POLIO					
OPV	2	02/18/1991	1	NE		NE	NE
		DTP					
DTaP	20	02/18/1991	1	NE		NE	NE
		MMR					
MMR	3	02/18/1993	1	NE		NE	NE
MMR	3	05/23/1995	2	NE		NE	NE
		HIB					
Hib	17	05/23/1995	1	NE		NE	NE
		HEP B					
Hep B-adol or ped	8	05/23/1995	1	NE		NE	NE

Care Plan

Name	CVX Code	Min Date	Max Date	Dose #
Hep B	45	08/25/2016	08/16/2090	2
Varicella	21	08/25/2016	08/15/2050	1
Influenza	88	08/25/2016	08/16/2090	1
Tdap	115	08/25/2016	08/16/2090	1
Zoster (shingles)	121	08/16/2050	08/16/2090	1
PCV13	133	08/16/2055	08/16/2090	1
PPV23	33	08/16/2056	08/16/2090	1

Figure 4.10   Human-readable display of an IC document.

of *merging* and *linking* correspond to the two subtly different approaches to de-duplication illustrated in Figures 4.2 and 4.3. The difference between a merge and a link is aptly described in the HL7 Version 2.5.1 standard. A merge is described as follows:

```
<component>
    <structuredBody classCode="DOCBODY" moodCode="EVN">
      <component>
        <section classCode="DOCSECT" moodCode="EVN">
          <templateId root="2.16.840.1.113883.10.20.1.6" />
          <templateId root="1.3.6.1.4.1.19376.1.5.3.1.3.23" />
          <id root="e30f8cc3-6af1-4bea-8e1a-29b813ca16fb" />
          <code code="11369-6" codeSystem="2.16.840.1.113883.6.1"
codeSystemName="LOINC" displayName="HISTORY OF IMMUNIZATIONS" />
          <title>Immunizations</title>
          <text mediaType="text/x-hl7-
text+xml"><table><thead><tr><td>Name</td><td>CVX Code</td><td>Date Admin</td><td>Dose
#</td><td>Mfg Code</td><td>Lot
Number</td><td>Route</td><td>Site</td></tr></thead><tbody><tr><td ID="ImmGroup-0"
align="center" colspan="8">POLIO</td></tr><tr><td ID="ImmName-93059507">OPV</td><td
ID="ImmCVX-93059507">2</td><td ID="ImmDateAdmin-93059507">02/18/1991</td><td
ID="ImmDoseNum-93059507">1</td><td ID="ImmMfgCode-93059507">NE</td><td
ID="ImmLotNumber-93059507"></td><td ID="ImmRoute-93059507">NE</td><td ID="ImmInj-
93059507">NE</td></tr><tr><td ID="ImmGroup-1" align="center"
colspan="8">DTP</td></tr><tr><td ID="ImmName-93059508">DTaP</td><td ID="ImmCVX-
93059508">20</td><td ID="ImmDateAdmin-93059508">02/18/1991</td><td ID="ImmDoseNum-
93059508">1</td><td ID="ImmMfgCode-93059508">NE</td><td ID="ImmLotNumber-
93059508"></td><td ID="ImmRoute-93059508">NE</td><td ID="ImmInj-
93059508">NE</td></tr><tr><td ID="ImmGroup-2" align="center"
colspan="8">MMR</td></tr><tr><td ID="ImmName-93059509">MMR</td><td ID="ImmCVX-
93059509">3</td><td ID="ImmDateAdmin-93059509">02/18/1993</td><td ID="ImmDoseNum-
93059509">1</td><td ID="ImmMfgCode-93059509">NE</td><td ID="ImmLotNumber-
93059509"></td><td ID="ImmRoute-93059509">NE</td><td ID="ImmInj-
93059509">NE</td></tr><tr><td ID="ImmName-93059510">MMR</td><td ID="ImmCVX-
93059510">3</td><td ID="ImmDateAdmin-93059510">05/23/1995</td><td ID="ImmDoseNum-
93059510">2</td><td ID="ImmMfgCode-93059510">NE</td><td ID="ImmLotNumber-
93059510"></td><td ID="ImmRoute-93059510">NE</td><td ID="ImmInj-
93059510">NE</td></tr><tr><td ID="ImmGroup-4" align="center"
colspan="8">HIB</td></tr><tr><td ID="ImmName-93059511">Hib </td><td ID="ImmCVX-
93059511">17</td><td ID="ImmDateAdmin-93059511">05/23/1995</td><td ID="ImmDoseNum-
93059511">1</td><td ID="ImmMfgCode-93059511">NE</td><td ID="ImmLotNumber-
93059511"></td><td ID="ImmRoute-93059511">NE</td><td ID="ImmInj-
93059511">NE</td></tr><tr><td ID="ImmGroup-5" align="center" colspan="8">HEP
B</td></tr><tr><td ID="ImmName-93059512">Hep B-adol or ped</td><td ID="ImmCVX-
93059512">8</td><td ID="ImmDateAdmin-93059512">05/23/1995</td><td ID="ImmDoseNum-
93059512">1</td><td ID="ImmMfgCode-93059512">NE</td><td ID="ImmLotNumber-
93059512"></td><td ID="ImmRoute-93059512">NE</td><td ID="ImmInj-
93059512">NE</td></tr></tbody></table></text>
```

Figure 4.11   IC document source code snippet.

A merge event signals that two distinct records have been combined together into a single record with a single set of identifiers and data surviving at the level of the merge. All records at a level subordinate to the merged identifier are combined under the surviving record.

Note: It is not the intent of the merge definition to define the application or implementation specifics of how various systems or environments define, use, or handle nonsurviving information. *Nonsurviving* in this document implies that a data set was existing

> in a fashion that was incorrect. Merging it into a new data set in itself implies that where there were two data sets, there is now only one. The means by which any system or environment conveys this new data set and the absence of the previous data set to the user is application specific. It is noted that some systems may still physically keep these "incorrect" data sets for audit trail or other purposes.*
>
> By contrast, a link is defined as linking two or more patients does not require the actual merging of patient information.… Following a link trigger event, sets of affected patient data records should remain distinct.†

Under a link, all records are deemed "correct." There is no incorrect, "nonsurviving" data.

By the time the IHE profiles were developed, the linked approach was generally embraced in the industry and embodied in what is known as a *master person index* (MPI). In IHE profiles, merging is reserved for situations in which a single system has been found to create two records for the same individual person—a true duplicate. A merge is used to combine their data elements and discard one of them.

The most important implication of a link versus a merge is that a link has an inverse operation, an *unlink*, that allows the link to be undone. A merge, on the other hand, is generally considered irreversible because of the unavailability of the nonsurviving data.

To illustrate the value of unlinking, consider a situation where the dates of birth in Figure 4.5 are applied to the Nat Young records in Figure 4.3. This is illustrated in Figure 4.12. It is now clear that the two records were previously linked in error. Whoever discovers the error first can now issue an unlink request. Rerunning the matching after unlinking will result in assigning new identifiers to the record, as in Figure 4.13.

Note in this example that the correction leads to changed immunization histories, including dose renumbering, for both patients, as now the records reflect only one MMR dose each. This in turn leads the decision support software to produce new recommendations. Instead of one patient who is up to date, there are now two patients, each needing an additional dose of MMR. Thus, the ability to unlink records and relink them has a direct impact on clinical decisions.

---

* Chapter 3, Section 3.6.2.
† Chapter 3, Section 3.6.3.

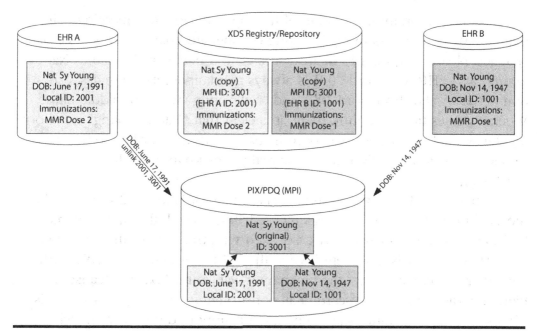

Figure 4.12   Before unlink.

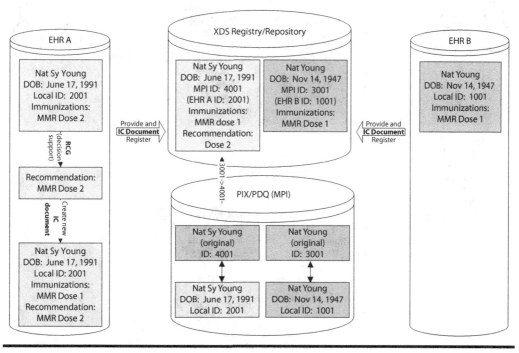

Figure 4.13   After unlink.

A second important implication of linking behavior over merging is in maintaining correctness in regenerating consolidated data when source data changes. Note in Figure 4.13 that the association between the name "Nat Sy Young" and EHR A's record 2001 is always maintained, as is the association between EHR B's record 1001 and "Nat Young" with no middle name. When it comes time to unlink them, it is clear that "Nat Sy Young" was born in 1991 while "Nat Young" was born in 1947. In fact, according to the data retrieved in Figure 4.7, "Nat Young" is really a nickname for "Robert Harold Nat Young."

By contrast, if the immunization registry user of Figure 4.2 were to add the 1947 birth date to Nat Young's merged 1001 record, the middle name "Sy" now becomes permanently associated with the 1947 birth date. Even if the matching error is discovered when the EHR user enters the 1991 birth date, there is no way to get the nickname "Nat Young" back, because the blank middle name was discarded as nonsurviving data (Figure 4.14). This is why unmerge operations are generally unsupported by record matching

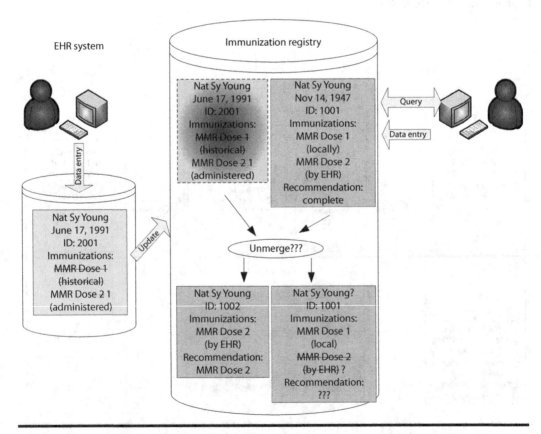

Figure 4.14   Updating a merged record.

standards. Incorrectly retaining the middle name "Sy" can lead to further matching errors when other records for the younger Nat Young arrive in the future.

Individual IHE Profiles

With the behavioral background of the IHE solution, let us now walk through the immunization profiles of Figure 4.8 and describe them individually.

Immunization Content and XDS

Recall the IC example of Figure 4.10 based on CDA. Documents conforming to all IHE content profiles including IC are managed by XDS. A single XDS Registry may be associated with more than one repository. A registry/repository deployment can manage documents described by content profiles that support a variety of healthcare domains—for example, medical summary documents. XDS also supports documents whose formats are undefined*; however, a content profile such as IC allows the communicating systems to request documents of particular types, to know how to display them, and to parse them if they wish and ingest their contents. By providing the XDS infrastructure to manage all kinds of healthcare documents, IHE supports the point-of-care requirement to gain a complete picture of a patient's records.

Figure 4.15, taken directly from the IHE Technical Framework, illustrates the roles and transactions of the XDS profile. The arrows labeled "ITI-8," "ITI-41," "ITI-42," and so on refer to transactions. Transactions are based on existing, or *base*, standards. The transactions of Figure 4.15 leverage a variety of base standards, including HL7 Version 2, HL7 Version 3, and non-HL7 standards—in particular, the ebXML standard of the Organization for the Advancement of Structured Information Standards (OASIS).

The boxes in Figure 4.15 indicate *roles*. IHE roles are an abstract notion, not to be confused with actual systems. That is, the six boxes of Figure 4.15 correspond to six roles, not to six systems. Each transaction includes both a sender and a receiver role. A single system may play either or both, but for a single transaction to be meaningful, two systems are implied.

---

* In other words, documents do not need to be based on CDA.

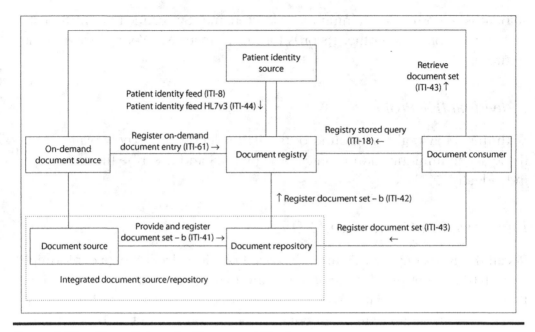

Figure 4.15   Cross-Enterprise Document Sharing.

A system playing the Document Registry role supplies information, or *metadata*, about the documents stored in the Document Repository and is used to locate documents on request. The Document Source provides the documents, and the Document Consumer retrieves them. In the deployment example of Figure 4.8, both EHR A and EHR B play the roles of Document Source and Document Consumer. The XDS Registry/Repository system plays both the roles of Document Registry and Document Repository. The MPI plays the role of Patient Identity Source. An On-Demand Document Source is a variation of a Document Source that is not depicted in Figure 4.8.

Because XDS is used for a variety of document types used in healthcare, the EHR generating the IC document may include other content sections, such as medications, lab results, problem lists, and so forth. The example IC document of Figure 4.10 includes a medications history that, as we shall see presently, can be used in immunization decision support.

PIX, PDQ, and Pediatric Demographics

As shown in Figure 4.8, XDS is meant to be used in conjunction with PIX and PDQ.

PIX includes a Cross-Reference Manager role that cross-references, or links, patient identifiers assigned by different *source* systems to the same individual person. PDQ includes a Patient Demographic Manager, which associates traits with identifiers, for the purpose of discovering existing records when identifiers are unknown. Because traits are also used in matching, PIX and PDQ are often implemented by the same system—an MPI. The MPI of Figure 4.8 plays both the roles of Cross-Reference Manager and Patient Demographics Manager, supporting both PIX and PDQ.

PIX and PDQ profile the HL7 Version 2 messages that are best suited to interacting with a "Cross-Reference Manager" or MPI.*

- The *Patient Identity Feed (ITI-8)* transaction constrains the HL7 Version 2.3.1 *admit, discharge, and transfer* (ADT) message to send new or updated patient records to the MPI.
- *Patient Identity Management* is very similar to Patient Identity Feed but is based on the 2.5.1 version of the HL7 base standard. It includes some additional data elements that are leveraged by Pediatric Demographics. Patient Identity Management also includes link and unlink operations (or *trigger events*), which Patient Identity Feed does not, although its base standard, HL7 Version 2.3.1, does.
- *PIX Query* obtains a list of identifiers that are cross-referenced with a given identifier.
- *PIX Update Notification* allows an MPI to keep interested systems updated as to its cross-referenced identifiers without having to query for them.
- The *Patient Demographics Query (ITI-21)* constrains the HL7 Version 2.5.1 Query by Parameter (QBP)† message to identify existing records for a patient when only his demographics are known.

The Patient Identity Feed transactions (ITI-8 or ITI-43) of Figure 4.15 provide the MPI identifier, called the *XAD-PID*, to the Document Registry of Figure 4.8. The XAD-PID used in XDS is not the same as the *local identifier* provided by to the MPI by the EHR systems. The intent of XDS is that the MPI will cross-reference the local identifiers, then provide its own, internal identifier, or XAD-PID, to XDS, one per individual person. The MPI receives the local identifiers from the EHRs via another instance of a Patient Identity Feed or via a Patient Identity Management (ITI-30) transaction.

---

* Technically, with a Patient Identifier Cross-Reference Manager; MPI is common language.
† QBP makes an appearance later in the successor version to the 2.3.1 guide, "HL7 Version 2.5.1 Implementation Guide for Immunization Messaging" or "2.5.1 Guide."

A difference between Patient Identity Management and Patient Identity Feed is that the former includes the requirement to support link and unlink operations. At the time of writing, PIX supports Patient Identity Management but XDS does not. The XAD-PID Change Management (XPID) profile, released for trial use in 2015, adds a transaction that supports unlinking and relinking. XPID adds the requirement to send local patient identifiers to XDS, in addition to the XAD-PID. The XPID profile, along with an IHE white paper entitled "XDS Patient Identity Management White Paper" that preceded it,* provides an elucidating discussion of the need for the relinking capability.

The EHR systems of Figure 4.8 supply, not their own local identifiers for Nat Young, but rather the XAD-PID generated by the MPI when providing or retrieving documents to/from the XDS Repository. To get the XAD-PID corresponding to the local identifier, one option, illustrated in our deployment example, is for each system to query the MPI using a PIX Query prior to accessing the XDS Repository. The EHR supplies its local identifier to the PIX Query as search criteria and gets back a list of cross-referenced identifiers, including the XAD-PID. The EHR then uses the XAD-PID—3001 in our deployment example—to either submit a document or retrieve a document set.

An alternative deployment is for the MPI to always keep each system whose identifiers it cross-references—that is, each system in its *affinity domain*—updated with the XAD-PID that corresponds to each of its local IDs using the PIX Update Notification transaction. This solution requires that all of the systems be correctly synchronized with any changes to the XAD-PID, such as those which may occur via link and unlink operations.

Pediatric Demographics is an *option* to PIX and PDQ[†] to enhance matching functionality when the patient database contains a preponderance of pediatric records, as is the case in immunization as well as certain other public health registries. An *option* is a feature of a transaction that is not required for basic conformance to a profile; rather, its implementation is "optional." Every year, IHE hosts a "Connectathon" at which system developers gather to test their conformance to profiles. So, for example, one Connectathon test for PIX may exclude the requirements of Pediatric Demographics, while another test includes it.

---

* http://www.ihe.net/Technical_Framework/upload/IHE_ITI_WhitePaper_Patient_ID_Management_Rev2-0_2011-03-04.pdf (March 4, 2011).
† For purposes of comparison, we focus on the HL7 Version 2 flavors of PIX and PDQ. IHE has special profiles for the HL7 Version 3 flavors of PIX and PDQ.

We previously touched on the particular difficulties of immunization registries in matching records belonging to pediatric twins and other multiple births. Pediatric Demographics adds data elements to the PIX and PDQ* pertaining to a child's birth and household:[†]

- Mother's Maiden Name
- Patient Home Telephone
- Patient Multiple Birth Indicator
- Patient Birth Order
- Last Update Date/Time
- Last Update Facility

A common mother's maiden name points to two records belonging to the same child. It can become misleading when their mother's maiden name, address, and date of birth cause two children who are twins to be mistaken for the same child, but a multiple birth indicator and birth order will distinguish the children in that case.

Last Update Date/Time and Last Update Facility are examples of traits used in matching that are not strictly demographic. Instead, they substitute for visit information.[‡] Provider visits on the same day point to two children brought to a doctor together rather than two records for the same child. Systems implementing the Pediatric Demographic option of PIX must support the *Patient Identity Management (ITI-30)* transaction, which is based on the HL7 Version 2.5.1 ADT message. Last Update Date/Time and Last Update Facility are not present in the earlier HL7 Version 2.3.1 ADT message.

Request for Clinical Guidance

The IHE RCG profile provides record consolidation and decision support functionality and completes the requirements of the immunization use case.

RCG is based on HL7 Version 3 messaging rather than CDA. Both Version 3 messaging and CDA derive from the HL7 Version 3 Reference Information Model (RIM), so they have similar structures and can store

---

* And PIXV3 and PDQV3.
[†] IHE, "IHE IT Infrastructure (ITI) Technical Framework, Volume 1 (ITI TF-1): Integration Profiles; Revision 12.0 Final Text," September 18, 2015, line 1402.
[‡] Visit information could also have been directly obtained by adding a *patient visit* segment to the ADT and QBP messages, but this would have been a complex change that would require more modification in field implementations, and so was rejected.

equivalent data elements. In our deployment example in Figure 4.8, EHR A uses RCG to process data elements extracted from the retrieved documents in order to inform the user of the vaccines due that day. The RCG service itself may be hosted by the local EHR, or it could be hosted elsewhere and accessed via the Internet. The EHR calling the RCG service can do whatever it needs to with the output: display it to a user, store it in its database, or convert it into a new document. A common workflow is to perform decision support once to recommend the vaccine due that day, give the vaccine, then run it again with the new vaccine included in order to validate and number the doses and recommend the next vaccine. This new recommendation could be included in the new document that the EHR submits to the XDS Repository for future retrieval by others. Note that the new document is now owned and authenticated by the EHR that created it, even if it was built on data that was extracted from documents created by other systems and retrieved from the XDS Repository.

Recall that the IC format supports more than just immunization information. The integrated patient information of the IC solution has direct implications for immunization decision support—the VFM. An insightful point made by a physician and key IHE contributor during the IHE discussions on IC was that the (additional) clinical detail contained in CDA is essential in computing the next vaccine recommendations. Vaccine schedules include shots that should be avoided, because they are *contraindicated*, as well as those that should be given. Certain vaccines may be contraindicated, for example, by immunodeficiency, a severe reaction to a previous vaccine, or pregnancy. A slight variation of a contraindication is a *precaution*—conditions that suggest a vaccine may be given, but with precautions. Finally, vaccines may be unnecessary if immunity can be presumed. Lab tests called *titers* or a certain disease history, such as a prior record of having chicken pox, may signal immunity. Avoiding a vaccine, if possible, not only saves money and time but also eliminates any risk, however small, of side effects or *adverse events*.

The IC format accommodates the medical record elements that flag these special cases. Some, such as disease history, might be called out directly; others, such as immunodeficiency, might need to be inferred. For example, a patient taking certain medications such as prednisone or chemotherapy drugs may be presumed to have a weakened immune system. Such medication records can be put to use by an immunization decision support service in flagging contraindications and precautions.

Such detail may need to be interpreted and reformatted prior to being supplied to an immunization registry system. Immunization registries are limited, both by mission and by law, in what clinical information they can store.* Certain generalized conditions, such as a previous anaphylactic (life-threatening) reaction to a vaccine or a history of a relevant disease such as chicken pox, may be stored when explicitly called out, but the detail from which such conditions are inferred is usually not allowed.

RCG offers the opportunity to pass in such detail without storing it and/ or for such a service to be deployed anywhere on the network that is convenient. Such a decision support service is considered *stateless*; that is, it does not store patient records or other information between invocations.† In fact, it does not even require the identity of the patient. Only the patient's immunization history, medical conditions, age, and (for some vaccines) gender are required as input.

Behavioral Analysis

Applied to the IHE profiles, Table 4.1 might be updated as follows.

Table 4.2 illustrates the inclusion in IHE profiles of the three advances discussed at the beginning of this chapter.

- Separation of concerns is seen in having different profiles for patient identification and clinical documents, and in the existence of a separate profile just for decision support.
- CDA principles of wholeness, stewardship, and potential for authentication are supported by the IC profile.
- Merges and links are explicitly supported in record matching.

Recall that the effort to include immunizations and public health in IHE profiles was motivated by a desire to facilitate interoperability between point-of-care EHR systems and public health. In developing its immunization profiles, IHE recognized that legacy immunization registry systems were based on the legacy 2.3.1 Guide, and that asking them to upgrade to support the PIX, PDQ, XDS, and RCG profiles might be unrealistic.‡ IHE broadly suggested that a middleware system such as an integration broker translate back

---

* There may also be cases where XDS repositories—for example, hosted by an HIE—can store immunization records that the immunization registry cannot—for example, if the source provider meets HIE consent requirements but not immunization registry requirements.
† That is, it does not store information but relies on the data passed in and out.
‡ The approach of building the IHE profiles on the 2.3.1 Guide was initially considered but ultimately rejected.

Table 4.2   IHE Immunization Profiles Behavioral Analysis

Data Exchange	
Query	For patient identification: PIX. For patient demographics: PDQ. For clinical content: XDS. IC documents provide a standard, CDA-based format for clinical data exchange.
Update	For patient identification: PIX. For patient demographics: PDQ. For clinical content: XDS. IC documents provide a standard, CDA-based format for clinical data exchange.
Match and Consolidate	
PIX and PDQ relate all the records for a patient by linking them. Both merge and link are supported. XDS may be used to request a set of documents related to one patient. Consolidation is deployment dependent; either the last system to submit an IC document must consolidate before providing it to XDS, or consolidation must be done on the fly by the requesting system.	
Decision Support	
RCG	

and forth between XDS and the messages of the 2.3.1 Guide. The details of the intermediary were not specified.

Intermediaries began to materialize when the Meaningful Use incentive program accelerated the adoption both of HL7 Version 2 public health messages and of IHE solutions. Since the Meaningful Use Stages 1 and 2 immunization registry reporting requirements included only VXUs from EHRs to immunization registries, and not queries, these first intermediaries implemented data flow in only one direction.

The deployment of Figure 4.16 is useful for providing copies of data to two user environments—IHE profiles and immunization registries—and allowing them to operate under the technical standards that are best suited to them. Because it is unidirectional, it cannot be said to demonstrate the integration of immunization registry data into the IHE-based picture of complete patient records in fulfillment of Figure 4.17. That challenge has yet to be met. As Meaningful Use moves into Stage 3 and requires queries, such intermediaries will be required to supply such services if the user is to receive an integrated vision of each patient's records. One can speculate that a possible future direction of mutual IHE and HL7 standards efforts will include the fleshing out of the intermediary of Figure 4.17.

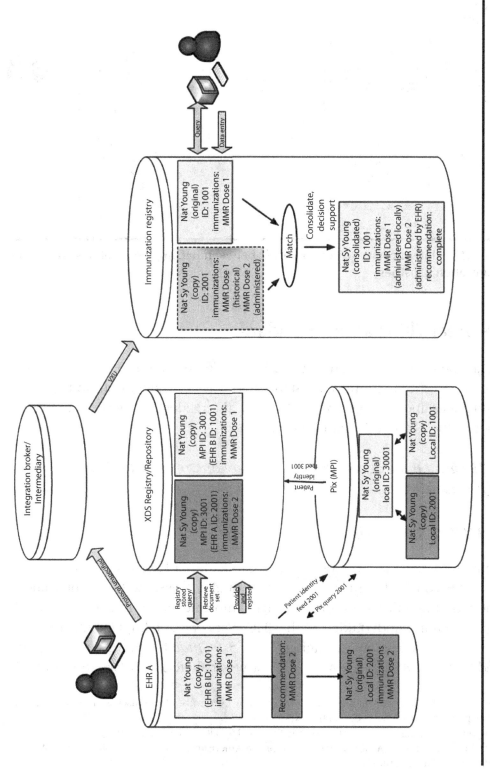

Figure 4.16   Meaningful Use Stages 1 and 2 intermediaries.

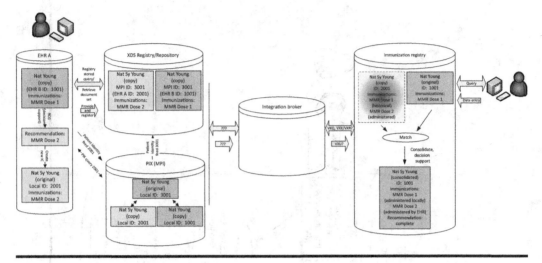

Figure 4.17   Intermediary to communicate between IHE implementations and legacy immunization registries.

The Great Thing about Standards

Even as the need to harmonize the 2.3.1 Guide and IHE profiles was being recognized, other immunization standards were emerging, both in the United States and internationally.* By now, the reader may appreciate the humor in the old joke in standards circles:

> *The great thing about standards is there are so many to choose from!*

The HL7 2.5.1 Guide

Meaningful Use included, not the 2.3.1 Guide, but a later version of it based on HL7 Version 2.5.1, which appeared at roughly the same time. Publication of the IHE immunization profiles for trial implementation in 2008 coincided roughly with the undertaking of the "HL7 Version 2.5.1 Implementation Guide for Immunization Messaging,"† or *2.5.1 Guide* for short, was first published by the CDC and AIRA‡ in 2010. It was balloted as *informative* in HL7

---

* Both HL7 and IHE are international organizations; however, most of the discussion in this chapter on this point is derived from US-centric experience.
† At the time of writing, the current version is Release 1.5, dated October 1, 2014.
‡ Not to be confused with ARRA, the acronym for the American Recovery and Reinvestment Act, which funded Meaningful Use.

through the HL7 Public Health and Emergency Response (PHER) workgroup that year. The primary objective was to upgrade from HL7 Version 2.3.1 to Version 2.5.1. Also scoped in were

- The expansion of detail in an effort to remove ambiguity
- Replacing the VXQ query message with the more general-purpose QBP query message*
- The correction of certain errors, including the failure, discussed in the 2.3.1 Guide "Message Set" section, to properly distinguish between an exact match and a single possible match in the response to a demographic query
- Other incremental improvements based on 15 years of immunization registry field experience

HL7 Version 3 Messaging

Development of the HL7 Version 3 Immunization Administration Topic (POIZ) was driven by representatives of Canada and Europe, where HL7 Version 3 messaging had strong governmental support.

POIZ offers several advances over Version 2. First, like the IHE profiles, it separates patient identification from immunization information exchange by relying on Version 3 messages designed for that purpose. Second, it includes an option to retrieve immunization records as a group, or *population*, of patients. Finally, it includes explicit queries for the next recommended vaccine or patient status, similar to IHE's RCG.

POIZ never achieved much uptake in the United States.

Service-Oriented Architecture Standards

The SOA standards arose from the momentum that emerged on the heels of general, non-healthcare web services technology. Much of the success of SOA is based on its emphasis on cost reduction through the reusability of services. It is unsurprising, then, that SOA support for immunizations derives

---

* Recall that QBP is used in the IHE Patient Demographic Query (PDQ) profile to retrieve patient identifiers by demographic search criteria. A different trigger event, however, is used. The 2.5.1 Guide uses a more general-purpose trigger event; PDQ makes use of the trigger events designed for interaction with an MPI. It is also interesting to note that the HL7 Version 2.5.1 base standard still supports the VXQ message, which is specific to immunizations; but the implementation guide chose to use something else: the QBP.

from general-purpose services that can be applied to any healthcare domain. Mirroring the broad immunization registry functions described previously, they include

- Identity Cross-Reference Service (IXS)
- Retrieve, Locate, and Update Service (RLUS)
- Decision Support Service (DSS)

The SOA standards were developed under the auspices of the Healthcare Services Specification Program (HSSP), a group of enterprise architects working collaboratively across the HL7 SOA Working Group, the Object Management Group (OMG), and IHE organizations. A parallel initiative at this time was SAIF, which was more of a theoretical approach to SOA development. Individual service specifications have been the domain of HSSP.

HSSP standards approach reusability by extracting the common elements of a service into an abstract portion of the service definition. It then allows for multiple *concrete* service definitions on different *platforms*—message, document, or service standards*—to be developed that conform to the abstract definition. To this end, HSSP standards consist of

- A *service-functional model*, developed by HL7, which describes the required functionality
- A *technical specification*, developed by OMG, which specifies the service interface, payload, and behavior

A technical specification in turn includes

- A *platform-independent model* (PIM), which describes the abstract, common elements
- One or more *platform-specific models* (PSMs), each rendering the service using a particular standard.

For example, a first RLUS PSM might make use of the VXU message of the 2.5.1 Guide, where a second PSM makes use of the IHE XDS standard and the IC profile.

---

* Strictly speaking, the PSM can be based on a proprietary format. Usually, the PSM is based on some standard.

Fast Healthcare Interoperability Resources

FHIR is the current focus of HL7. Driven by Australian and Canadian HL7 members, a motivation of FHIR is ease of implementation, particularly compared with HL7 Version 3, which carries a great deal of modeling information on the line protocol. The following is from the FHIR executive summary.[*]

FHIR offers many improvements over existing standards:

- A strong focus on implementation—fast and easy to implement (multiple developers have had simple interfaces working in a single day)
- Multiple implementation libraries, many examples available to kick-start development
- Specification is free for use with no restrictions
- Interoperability out-of-the-box—base resources can be used as is, but can also be adapted for local requirements
- Evolutionary development path from HL7 Version 2 and CDA—standards can co-exist and leverage each other
- Strong foundation in web standards—XML, JSON, HTTP, OAuth, etc.
- Support for RESTful architectures and also seamless exchange of information using messages or documents
- Concise and easily understood specifications
- A human-readable wire format for ease of use by developers
- Solid ontology-based analysis with a rigorous formal mapping for correctness

FHIR includes Immunization[†] and Immunization Recommendation[‡] resources, both of which are considered at the time of writing to be at Maturity Level 1 on a scale of 0 to 5, where 5 indicates the most mature standards.[§] FHIR continues the modern trend of separating Patient and Immunization resources and providing human-readable text fallback "for clinical safety."[¶] The structure of the FHIR Immunization resource was carefully harmonized with the 2.5.1 Guide and POIZ by the PHER group, which manages both those standards within HL7.

---

[*] https://www.hl7.org/fhir/summary.html.
[†] https://www.hl7.org/fhir/immunization.html.
[‡] https://www.hl7.org/fhir/immunizationrecommendation.html.
[§] https://www.hl7.org/fhir/resource.html#maturity.
[¶] https://www.hl7.org/fhir/summary.html.

The FHIR website discusses the likelihood of disruption in the near future of healthcare technology—a good segue for our concluding remarks and anticipation of the future.

Behavioral Analysis

Table 4.3 lists the specific messages, documents, services, and profiles, collectively referred to as *artifacts*, used by all the standards discussed in this chapter to implement the primary behaviors required by the immunization use case: data exchange, record matching and consolidation, and decision support. Detailed discussion of how each artifact implements these behaviors is out of scope to this discussion; nevertheless, the trend toward the separation of concerns can be observed. POIZ, SOA, and FHIR each specify different artifacts for each primary behavior, including a separate decision support standard, and scoping out and/or the reuse of standards for such behaviors as matching and consolidation across multiple healthcare domains. These standards appeared simultaneous to or after the IHE profiles, at a time when the need for linking and unlinking and patient-centric data were already well understood. As such, these standards are more like the IHE profiles in the behaviors they support.

Table 4.3   Artifacts by Behavior of Multiple Immunization Standards

HL7 V2.3.1	IHE profiles	HL7 V2.5.1	POIZ	SOA	FHIR Resource
Data Exchange					
VXU, VXQ	XDS/IC	VXU, QBP	Various	RLUS	Immunization
Match and Consolidate					
VXU, VXQ	PIX and PDQ	VXU, QBP	Out of scope	IXS	Patient
Decision Support					
VXQ	RCG	QBP	Patient immunization status requested	DSS	Immunization Recommendation

Conclusion

Immunization standards provide an excellent case study for recognizing the need for behavioral specification and developing a systematic method of doing so. The specification of behavior in standards is a new topic that is still in its infancy. Much work remains to be done in this area of standards development.

As systems progress in their ability to support the advanced behaviors discussed in this chapter, the immunization use case itself may evolve, as software support for users becomes more capable and more available. Opportunities for the evolution of the use case as supported by the standards already described in this chapter include

- Patient involvement in verifying that the records that have been linked to them truly are their records
- Direct patient reminders that their vaccines are due
- The ability to use the full medical record in flagging vaccine contraindications and precautions

Chapter 5

Bumrungrad International Hospital Implementation of the Patient Plan of Care Profile in Bangkok, Thailand

Luann Whittenburg, Jiraporn Lekdumrongsak,
Aunchisa Meetim, and Amornrat Klaikaew

Nursing practice makes a difference.

Virginia K. Saba
Pioneer of computer technology in nursing

Contents

Background

The Patient Plan of Care (PPOC) Profile addresses an urgent global call to reduce healthcare fragmentation and expand the interoperability of healthcare data. The PPOC was developed by Integrating the Healthcare Enterprise (IHE), an initiative of healthcare professionals and the industry to improve how computer systems share healthcare information. "IHE Profiles help care providers use information more effectively for optimal patient care" (IHE, 2014). IHE Profile data exchanges relate to creating and managing individualized patient care, and "systems that implement integration profiles solve interoperability problems" (IHE, 2016). The PPOC data exchange process is known as the *coordination of care* and is clinically viewed as a process of active, cooperative engagement between patients and care teams toward a shared healthcare goal (American Academy of Family Physicians, 2015). Within healthcare information management, the coordination of care is a process involving the exchange of coded, patient information and data across providers, types and levels of service, sites of care, and timeframes (Schlossman, 2013).

From similar definitions, the American Nurses Association (ANA) reflects, "Nurses are the primary coordinators of patient care and act as healthcare advocates for individuals, families, communities, and populations" (ANA, 2012). At present, nursing information documentation of a patient's response to an actual or potential health threat is rarely electronically transferred between and among healthcare information record systems. Recently, there have been efforts to define healthcare data standards related to quality, cost, patient safety, continuity of care, and the translation of clinical research findings to the bedside (Richesson and Krisher, 2007). These data standards focus on enabling data exchange, portability, and reusability (Chalmers, 2006). Yet, in most healthcare settings (e.g., outpatient and emergency care; primary care; inpatient, procedural, rehabilitation, and subacute facilities), nurses manage the continuity of care and the movement of patients. Nurses address what is the most important "care" at a specific moment in a given situation and what patient care is expected to happen next (Ebright, 2010). Researchers often report teamwork as an essential component for best practice in clinical settings (Institute of Medicine [IOM], 2001) and note that the effectiveness and efficiency of the team depends on members having up-to-date information and situational awareness (Endsley, 1995). In this context, the data collection of patient assessment information and knowledge of the complexity of care performed by nurses is one of the largest data gaps in worldwide health-care systems.

Within nursing practice, patient care collaboration between patients and families and every nurse is integral to patient care quality and the efficient use of healthcare resources (ANA, 2012).

> Patient-centered care is a core professional standard and compe-
> tency for nursing practice and essential component of the care
> coordination process to improve patient care outcomes, facilitate
> effective interprofessional collaboration, and to decrease health-
> care costs across patient populations and health care settings.
> (ANA, 2016, p. 1)

Atherly and Thorpe (2011) demonstrated significant cost reductions among high-cost, chronically ill patients by using an interprofessional team and nurse care coordinators to educate and empower patients in self-care activities. Registered nurse care coordinators worked with patients to pro-mote adherence to care plans. The research demonstrated that "total annual costs for participants were 15.7% lower than for the control group. A descrip-tive analysis found the mean spending for the intervention group was lower than for the control group" (Atherly and Thorpe, 2011, p. 9).

Research by Marek et al. (2010) demonstrated the continuity-of-care coordination by nurses decreased the overall costs for a geriatric Medicare/Medicaid population in a community-based long-term care program. The study purpose was to examine the relationship of nurse care coordination (NCC) to the costs of Medicare/Medicaid in a community-based care pro-gram called Missouri Care Options (MCO). A retrospective cohort design compared 57 MCO clients with NCC with 80 MCO clients without NCC. The program's total cost was measured using Medicare and Medicaid claims data-bases. A fixed effects analysis was used to estimate the relationship of the NCC intervention to costs. In controlling for high resource use on admission, the study found that monthly Medicare costs lowered within 12 months of NCC interventions. And nurse care coordinators followed these older adults across all care settings.

In the United States, healthcare access is characterized by overuse, underuse, and misuse with unsustainable costs and suboptimal outcomes (Orszag, 2008). The "Healthcare Imperative: Lowering Costs and Improving Outcomes" (IOM, 2011) report found patient populations who received healthcare services wasted an estimated $240 billion annually due to *uncoordinated care.* The report identified uncoordinated care in the use of inappropriate combinations of prescriptions and therapeutically duplicative drugs, a lack of adherence to prescribed treatment plans, duplicative diagnostic services, care services provided by multiple providers and pharmacies, emergency visits for nonemergency care, and other services, which represented "on average 10% of patients … approximately 45% of drug costs, 30% of medical costs, and 35% of total health care costs … annually" (Owen, 2011, p. 4). Uncoordinated care was reported at an average annual cost of care five times higher than other care and could translate into an estimated cumulative potential savings of over $2 trillion by 2018 with better coordinated care (IOM, 2011).

The PPOC describes the content structures for managing patient care using a plan of care based on the data elements from the ANA Nursing Process to reduce care fragmentation and individualize the coordination of care. The PPOC specifies Health Level Seven International (HL7) Clinical Document Architecture (CDA) to represent the content structures of the ANA Nursing Process: Assessment, Diagnosis, Outcomes Identification, Planning, Implementation, and Evaluation data elements along with IHE Cross-Document Sharing (XDS), Cross-Enterprise Document Sharing (XDS), Cross-Enterprise Document Reliable Interchange (XDR), and Cross-Enterprise Document Media Interchange (XDM) bindings. These IHE Profiles provide a mechanism for the electronic exchange of data related to creating and managing individualized patient care between and among health information technology (HIT) and health information record systems (HIRS). The mission of IHE Patient Care Coordination (PCC) Profiles are to support the coordination of care for patients where care crosses providers, patient conditions and health concerns, or time. The PPOC was developed to support the exchange of patient care data by nurses in a standard framework for PCC supported by the ANA Nursing Process using coded, standardized nursing terminology; the Clinical Care Classification (CCC) System, named as the first national nursing terminology standard by the Department of Health and Human Services (Saba, 2007).

The CCC System is a research-based, coded terminology standard that identifies the discrete data elements of nursing practice, the *essence of care.* The CCC System includes a holistic framework and coding structure of nursing diagnoses, interventions, and outcomes for assessing, documenting, and classifying care in all healthcare settings (CCC, n.d.). The CCC System research study was conducted under a federal contract with the Health Care Financing Agency (HCFA), now the Centers for Medicare and Medicaid Services, "to develop and demonstrate a method for classifying patients to predict resources and measure outcomes" (Saba, 2012, p. 7).

The CCC structure consists of two interrelated terminologies, the CCC of Nursing Diagnoses and Outcomes and the CCC of Nursing Interventions/ Actions, organized into a single system categorized by 21 Care Components representing the functional, physiological, psychological, and health behavioral patterns of care. The CCC links the diagnoses, interventions, and outcomes to each other and enables these to be mapped to other health-related terminologies. The coding uses a "five-character alphanumeric structure ... based on the format of the *International Statistical Classification of Disease and Related Health Problems: Tenth Revision (ICD-10)* specifically designed for computer processing" (Saba, 2012, p. 88).

The 21 Care Components of the CCC provide a standardized framework and "correlate with the first standard of the nursing process—**Assessment** of the patients' signs and symptoms" (Figure 5.1). The CCC of Nursing Diagnoses and Outcomes consists of 176 concepts (60 major categories and 116 subcategories) representing concrete patient problems. "The **Diagnosis** is a granular atomic-level diagnostic condition based on the analysis and synthesis of the assessed signs and systems, Care Components, and problems that require therapeutic nursing care to alter the health status of the patient" (Saba, 2012, p. 89).

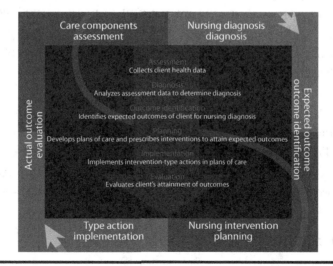

Figure 5.1 **Nursing process and CCC diagram. (From Saba, V.K., "Clinical Care Classification System," brochure, Arlington, VA: SabaCare, 2004. Reprinted with permission.)**

The expected outcomes represent the goals of nursing care [and] are identified by three nursing outcome qualifiers that maximize the **Outcome Identification** from the 176 Nursing Diagnoses to 528 Expected Outcomes. Each Nursing Diagnosis requires an Expected Outcome to achieve a measureable outcome resulting from the therapeutic nursing care that alters the health status of the patient. Three qualifiers are presented in the present tense:

- *Improve or Resolve* the patient's condition
- *Stabilize or Maintain* the patient's condition
- *Support the Deterioration* of the patient's condition (Saba, 2012, p. 89)

> The CCC of Nursing Interventions consists of 201 interventions (77 core categories and 124 subcategories). Nursing Interventions are granular atomic-level services or core concepts used for *Planning* and describing the proposed Plan of Care (POC) for the patient. The Four Action Types—Assess, Perform, Teach, and Manage— enhance the 201 interventions to 804 interventions/actions. Each Nursing Intervention requires an Action Type qualifier. The Action Type qualifier focuses on the specific action needed for the **Implementation** of each of the Nursing Interventions in the POC. The Action Types provide the measures used to determine the status of the care process at any given point in time as well as identify nursing workload, resources, and the nursing cost of patient care. With the nursing interventions, the Action Types provide the evidence for clinical decision-making. (Saba, 2012, p. 89)

In the CCC, Actual Outcomes are also identified by the same three qualifiers used to determine whether patient care goals were met or not met. "Each Nursing Diagnosis requires an Actual Outcome as an **Evaluation** of the therapeutic care or Nursing Intervention/Actions…. The Actual Outcomes qualifiers are presented in the past tense" (Saba, 2012, pp. 89–90).

CCC Example: Patient Has Difficulty Walking

Nursing Diagnosis and Outcome Coding:
Assessment: Activity Component (A)
Nursing Diagnosis: Physical Mobility Impairment (A01.5)

Expected Outcome (Goal): **Improve** Physical Mobility Impairment
(A01.5.**1**)
Actual Outcome: Physical Mobility Impairment **Improved** (A01.5.**1**)

Nursing Intervention/Actions Coding:
Component: Activity Component (A)
Nursing Intervention: Ambulation Therapy (A03.1)
Action Type: **Teach** Ambulation Therapy (A03.1.**3**) (Saba, 2012, p. 90)

Note: CCC Nursing Interventions do not exist without a Nursing Diagnosis. Without a Nursing Diagnosis, there is no logic for implementing a Nursing Intervention following the Nursing Process.

The US Department of Health and Human Services (HHS), Strategic Objective B, identifies care coordination as an essential healthcare strategy to control costs while achieving value in healthcare. In 2007, the CCC was adopted by HHS as the first national nursing standard recommended by the Healthcare Information Technology Standards Panel (HITSP) for electronic health records (EHRs) (HITSP, 2009a; US HHS 73 FR 3973, January 23, 2008).

The CCC uses the six standards of the ANA Nursing Process to describe nursing practice in a coding structure designed for retrieving data from computer information systems (Hardiker et al., 2002). The following section discusses the PPOC environment for use in the electronic nursing documentation system project at Bumrungrad International Hospital in Bangkok, Thailand.

Project Introduction and Implementation Environment

Bumrungrad International Hospital is an accredited Joint Commission International (JCI) multispecialty hospital located in the heart of Bangkok, Thailand. Founded in 1980, Bumrungrad is the first Asian hospital accredited by JCI, the international arm of the Joint Commission organization that reviews and accredits hospitals in the United States. Bumrungrad International is one of the largest private hospitals in Southeast Asia, with 580 beds and over 30 specialty centers offering state-of-the-art diagnostic, therapeutic, and intensive care facilities serving 1.1 million patients annually, including over 520,000 international patients (Bumrungrad, 2015).

In October 2009, the PPOC implementation project began with the index-ing of nursing data element requirements into a standard nursing terminol-ogy. The CCC was selected for data modeling because it describes, in an integrated, coded, standardized framework, nursing data for the exchange of care outcomes, continuity of care, and nursing services, and enables nurs-ing care visibility in electronic healthcare databases and records. An original *enterprise architecture* (EA) methodology was developed specifically for the implementation of the CCC in a clinical knowledge base (Goltra, 1978). The purpose was to index the nursing terminology to the full array of terminol-ogy standards and concepts in MEDCIN® with Intelligent Prompting™, allowing for the presentation, and documentation, of relevant clinical symp-toms, history, physical findings, and diagnoses to the CCC System from virtually any clinical condition. At the point of care, the method used the MEDCIN diagnostic index to focus on CCC Nursing Diagnoses using clinical diagnoses or signs and symptoms in patient documentation for aggregated data analysis.

In December 2012, the Bumrungrad International Nursing Informatics (NI) project team initiated the implementation of coded nursing documenta-tion using MEDCIN findings carrying a CCC code. The team used the CCC Information Model and ANA Nursing Process to integrate nursing concepts with MEDCIN findings (clinical terms) to establish an interoperable care plan generated from patient data collected by nurses at the bedside. There were 117 paper documents used by nurses to record patient assessments and nurs-ing care on diverse wards, such as medical, surgical, coronary care, intensive care, pediatrics, transplants, oncology, emergency departments, labor and delivery, dialysis, operating rooms, and education. As paper patient docu-mentation was complete, the document was scanned and a copy stored in digital format. The conversion process provided patient data for nursing care continuity. Scanning was labor intensive and time-consuming and the uncoded data was not suitable for care outcomes analysis. In February 2013, the nursing data element analysis began using a standardized worksheet to prepopulate each assessment concept from the nursing documents. There were approximately 9000 nursing data elements analyzed. The number of data elements per document ranged from 3 to 350. Each worksheet included a field for the collection of data element type: Text, Value, Y/N, Onset, and so on, as well as preassigned data properties, such as *history of, educa-tion of, moderate amount of,* and so on. Once a worksheet was populated, each nursing data element was reviewed and assigned to a MEDCIN find-ing based on semantic agreement using the International Organization for

Standardization (ISO) Degrees of Equivalence (ISO, 2010). Each semantic match for each nursing data element and MEDCIN finding was independently validated for reliability to prepare the implementation environment for the next steps.

In January 2013, Bumrungrad International executives identified electronic nursing documentation as an organizational priority and approved standardized nursing assessment documentation as the "next step" toward integrated physician–nurse documentation. Initial planning identified the essential documents for implementation. Of the 117 documents, 40 documents met 99.82% of the nursing documentation requirements. In the PPOC, nursing assessment documentation moved nurses from a traditional role as data collectors to a role as data consumers and highlighted the value of nurses to the organizational mission of providing high-level continuity of care and coordination.

Implementation nursing requirements

1. Electronic documentation must follow the Nursing Process.
2. Documentation must cover the full range of nursing care—that is, assessment, performance of care, teaching, and managing care as an interprofessional team.
3. Implement a recognized nursing information framework and terminology.
4. Implement a standards-based approach and process for implementation.

Implementation environment objectives

1. Expand nursing time for bedside patient care.
2. Reduce data redundancy in documentation.
3. Improve hand-off communication.
4. Increase satisfaction by decreased documentation time and improved readability.
5. Support nurse decision-making.
6. Ensure consistent application of nursing policies, procedures, and clinical practice guidelines.
7. Prepare for evolving documentation requirements from risk management, standards of practice, and external regulatory agencies.

Bumrungrad International chief nursing officer, Jiraporn Lekdumrongsak, RN, brought professional nurses together from various nursing practice areas and roles to contribute to the requirements for the electronic nursing documentation project. Nurses were the key decision-makers throughout the project life cycle and actively framed the functional and operational system requirements. System requirements from Amornrat Klaikaew, RN, principle solution specialist, and Aunchisa Meetim, RN, senior nurse manager, NI, and professional project management addressed the expectations of stakeholders through comprehensive project planning and execution. The Bumrungrad Nursing Center directors and the Nursing eDocumentation Council contributed expertise in the development of documentation system requirements for the implementation environment. A specific characteristic of the project was the remarkable level of effective communication among stakeholders for deliverables. The exceptional communication and monitoring of scope ensured the overall goals, schedules, and benefits of the project were producing the products, services, and results the project was undertaken to produce.

Selecting and Writing the Technical Specification

In 2008, IHE PCC Technical Committee approved the development of a Coded Nursing Documentation (CND) Profile (IHE, 2008) to describe content structures for a PPOC within IHE's technical framework. From 2008 to 2009, the IHE PCC Nursing Subcommittee began biweekly meetings to develop the profile, subsequently titled the Patient Plan of Care. The profile content authors were Saba and Whittenburg (2008) along with informatics nurse specialists, who convened to pinpoint the urgent need for nursing data interoperability in the standards development organization (SDO) community by the single largest group of healthcare professionals—nurses!

In 2009, the IHE PCC released the PPOC for public comment. The same year, the Office of the National Coordinator for Health Information Technology (ONC) initiated the development of clinical use cases to define the interoperability requirements for high-priority healthcare data through the Healthcare Information Technology Standards Panel (HITSP), a strategic partnership established through a contract with HHS and the American National Standards Institute (ANSI), which was selected to administer HITSP. One HITSP objective was to enable and advance the interoperability of healthcare applications and the interchanging of healthcare data to assure accurate use, access, privacy, and security to support both the delivery of care and public health (HITSP, 2009b). Separately, in June 2009, the PPOC was approved by the IHE PCC as a technical guideline and released as an electronic PPOC technical supplement for trial use. The PPOC is a practical solution to improve healthcare information exchange through the organized implementation of interoperable, structured, coded nursing POCs for PCC and safety.

In January 2011, the next phase of interoperability specifications occurred with the ONC launch of the Standards and Interoperability (S&I) Framework collaboration, a "community formed with participants from public and private sector experts in healthcare to collaborate on the interoperability challenges of the functional exchange of health information" (S&I, 2015). In the S&I definition by the Longitudinal Coordination of Care (LLC) workgroup, a care plan "represents the synthesis and reconciliation of multiple plans of care produced by each provider to address specific health concerns. It serves as a blueprint shared by all participants to guide the individual's care. As such, it provides the structure required to coordinate care across multiple sites, providers and episodes of care" (S&I, 2012, p. 2). In 2013, the LCC included "a consensus-driven dynamic plan that represents all of a patient's and care team members' prioritized concerns, goals, and planned interventions" (S&I, 2013, p. 6). In the Federal Health Information Model (FHIM) definition,

> A care plan is a planning and coordination tool to assist in delivery of integrated/collaborative care by a healthcare team within which the patient is the center of the team. A care plan supports the inclusion of health concerns and risks, health goals, care preferences and barriers, interventions, and iterative reviews during the planning and implementation phases of collaborative care. The care plan also supports communication of the whole, or parts of the plan, acceptance (or not) of the plan, and synchronization or reconciliation of multiple plans. (FHIM, n.d.)

From the Health Information and Management Systems Society's (HIMSS) *Dictionary of Healthcare Information Technology Terms, Acronyms and Organizations* (third edition), the PPOC definition is

1. A roadmap to guide all services that are involved with a patient's care. The plan of care contains goals or outcomes related to treatment options.
2. Based on the six steps/standards of the Nursing Process. (Whittenburg, 2013, p. 101)

According to HIMSS, a plan of care "may include patient-specific policies and procedures, protocols, clinical practice guidelines, clinical paths, care maps, or a combination thereof, to guide the format of the plan in some organizations. A care plan may include care, treatment, habilitation, and rehabilitation" (Whittenburg, 2013, p. 106).

In the Health Information Technology for Economic and Clinical Health (HITECH) Act, a component of the American Recovery and Reinvestment Act of 2009 (ARRA), there was a substantial commitment of US federal resources for widespread adoption of EHRs and "efficient, effective decisions about patient care through the improved aggregation, analysis, and communication of patient information, clinical alerts and reminders including support for diagnostic and therapeutic decisions" (ARRA, 2009; ONC, 2015a, 2015b). The PPOC was designed to standardize EHR communication and support the availability of patient data for nursing diagnostic and therapeutic decisions in a care plan that improves data aggregation through the following (IHE, 2009; Burns et al., 2014):

1. Standardize a systematic method for the digital exchange of data related to creating and managing patient plans of care across and between HIRS.
2. Enhance standardized Care Plan data interoperability using the ANA Nursing Process and CCC Information Model; vital professional nursing information frameworks.
3. Define Care Plan section structures for Clinical Document Architecture (CDA) documents from American National Standards Institute, Health Level Seven (HL7).
4. Define Care Plan content structures for the IHE Cross-Enterprise Document Sharing (XDS), Cross-Enterprise Document Reliable Interchange (XDR), and Cross-Enterprise Document Media Interchange (XDM) bindings as well as other IHE Integration Profiles such as the Patient Identifier Cross-Reference (PIX), Patient Demographic Query (PDQ), and the Notification of the Availability of documents (NAV). All the IHE Profiles (above) support security and privacy through the IHE Consistent Time (CT) and Audit Trail and the Node Authentication (ATNA) IHE Profiles.
5. Standardize collaboration with multiple healthcare disciplines—for example, primary care, emergency departments, ambulatory, outpatient, and inpatient services (psychiatric, residential addiction, and medical-surgical)—to reduce disparities in health outcomes.

6. Supports the coordination of care for patient population management to reduce overuse, underuse, and misuse in
   a. Emergency department visits
   b. Inpatient re-admissions
   c. Patient satisfaction and confidence in self-care management
   d. Patient safety during transition from an acute care to the home
   e. Improved clinical outcomes

"There are two actors in the PPOC Profile, the Content Creator and the Content Consumer. Content is generated by a Content Creator and consumed by a Content Consumer" (IHE, 2009, p. 10) (Figure 5.2). "The sharing or transmission of content from one actor to the other is addressed by the appropriate use of IHE Profiles" (IHE, p. 10) as previously described, including, but not limited to, XDS, XDR, XDM, PIX, and PDQ. "The sharing or transmission of content or updates from one actor to the other is addressed by the use of the PPOC as a content profile that is intended to eventually sit within a larger structure that contains documents related to the interdisciplinary continuity of care for the patient" (IHE, p. 4).

The PPOC defines the data elements for care planning along with the IHE bindings to support the exchange of information. Often health information record systems (HIRS) use a reference terminology for patient assessment documentation without an interactive plan of care for coordination. The effect diminishes the documentation of nursing assessment content conformance and continuity of care in the patient's integrated healthcare treatment

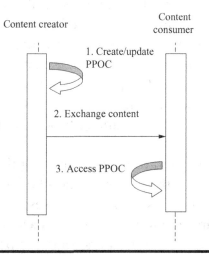

Figure 5.2 PPOC process flow. (From IHE International, IHE PCC, PPOC Rev. 1.0, 2009-05-2901, 2009.)

plan. With the use of the PPOC profile, content can be exchanged electronically between and among HIRS for each of the six steps of the Nursing Process. The PPOC content may also be exchanged with others who may update and return the PPOC to the sender, primary care provider, patient, and/or other interested parties such as disease managers, case managers, and care managers.

The process flow diagram in Figure 5.2 shows the movement of the PPOC over the course of care for a patient as an inpatient on a nursing ward. This diagram specifically excludes other infrastructure interactions for simplicity and readability. These infrastructure interactions may be found elsewhere in the PPOC and other IHE frameworks. (IHE, 2009, p. 14)

In 2012, the Use Care implementation of the PPOC technical supplement for trial use required a deeper technical understanding of the ANA Nursing Process. The PPOC contains a universal level of ANA Nursing Process competency, as described in Table 5.1. The components of the Nursing Process are also shown in the PPOC model (Figure 5.3).

The Nursing Process is the common thread uniting national and international professional nurses—the "essential core of *nursing* practice" (ANA, 2015b). The Nursing Process encompasses all significant actions taken by registered nurses and forms the "foundation of the nurse's decision making" (ANA, 2010, p. 17). When a patient arrives for care (e.g., upon admission or transfer of care) the patient receives an initial nursing assessment. In the care planning process, the nursing assessment determines the nursing diagnoses, outcomes identification (goals), and the planning of care with the patient or their advocate. The Nursing Process continues with the nurse providing care. This results in actions performed to care for the patient, followed by evaluation of the patient progress against the expected outcomes. Evaluation measures the current patient progress against the expected outcomes through subsequent assessments. These assessments are then used to adjust the Nursing Process. These components are performed continuously through the Nursing Process at macro- and micro-levels (IHE, 2009, p. 5).

Both the patient's status and the effectiveness of the nursing care must be continuously evaluated, and the care plan modified as needed (ANA, 2015b).

The Nursing Process requires a continual assessment and evaluation of patient responses to nursing interventions to achieve the identified nursing outcomes (Saba, 2007), and a "cyclical and ongoing process" with essentially no end until the patient's healthcare needs are met (Kozier et al., 2004, p. 261) (Table 5.2).

Table 5.1 Six Standards of the Nursing Process

Standard 1: Assessment
Definition: "Comprehensive data pertinent to the patient's health or the situation" (IHE, 2011, p. 14).
The first standard in delivering nursing care. "Nursing assessment includes not only physiological data, but also psychological, sociocultural, spiritual, economic, and lifestyle factors as well. For example, a nurse's assessment of a hospitalized patient in pain includes not only the physical causes and manifestations of pain, but the patient's response—an inability to get out of bed, refusal to eat, withdraw from family members, anger directed at hospital staff, fear, or request for more pain medication" (ANA, 2015b).
Standard 2: Diagnosis
Definition: Analysis of assessment data to determine the diagnoses or issues.
The nursing diagnosis is the nurse's clinical judgment about the client's response to actual or potential health conditions or needs. The diagnosis is the basis for the nurse's care plan (ANA, 2015b). A diagnosis may reflect not only that the patient is in pain, but that the pain has caused other problems such as anxiety, poor nutrition, and conflict within the family, or has the potential to cause complications; for example, respiratory infection is a potential hazard to an immobilized patient (ANA, 2015b).
Standard 3: Outcomes Identification
Definition: Expected outcomes individualized to the patient and situation (Saba, 2012).
"Based on the assessment and diagnosis, the nurse sets measurable and achievable short- and long-range goals for the patient. Assessment data, diagnosis, and goals are written in the patient's care plan so that nurses as well as other health professionals caring for the patient have access to it" (ANA, 2015b).
Standard 4: Planning
Definition: Development of prescribed strategies and alternatives to attain expected outcomes (Saba, 2012).
"Based on the measurable and achievable short- and long-range goals, planning may include moving from bed to chair at least three times per day (TID); maintaining adequate nutrition by eating smaller, more frequent meals; resolving conflict through counseling, or managing pain through adequate medication" (ANA, 2015b).
Standard 5: Implementation
Definition: Implementation of the identified care plan (Saba, 2012).
"Nursing care is implemented according to the care plan, so continuity of care for the patient during hospitalization and in preparation for discharge needs to be assured. Care is documented in the patient's record" (ANA, 2015b).
Standard 6: Evaluation
Definition: Evaluate the progress toward attainment of outcomes (IHE, 2011, p. 15).

Integrating the Healthcare Enterprise (IHE) Patient Plan of Care (PPOC) profile model, 2009

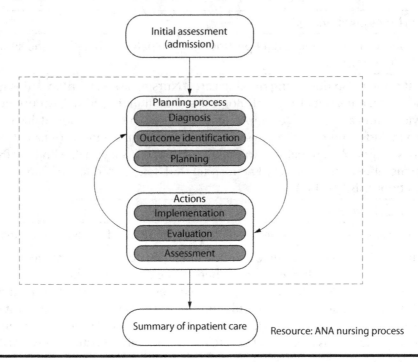

Figure 5.3 PPOC model. (From IHE International, IHE PCC, PPOC Rev. 1.0, 2009-05-2901, 2009.)

Table 5.2 Nursing Process Focus

• Patient-centered: Focused on patient care; adapted to meet needs/concerns.
• Goal-oriented: Interventions are determined by the nursing diagnoses and chosen for the purpose of achieving the nursing outcome.
• Universally applicable: Appropriate for any patient, of any age, with any clinical diagnosis, at any point on the health continuum and in any setting (e.g., school, clinic, hospital, or home) and across all nurse specialties (e.g., hospice, maternity, pediatric, etc.).
• Cognitive process: Involves nursing judgment and decision-making. The nurse is required to apply nursing knowledge systematically and logically to interpret, analyze, and use data to determine the appropriate plan of care based on knowledge of the physical, biological, and behavioral sciences. As part of academic preparation, nurses have biochemistry, biophysics, microbiology, anatomy, physiology, psychology, and sociology courses. This basic knowledge of the sciences enables nurses to recognize patient problems and determine how the patient's health is disrupted by a health problem.

PPOC Steps for Following the Nursing Process

1. A patient admitted as an inpatient to a hospital for a clinical diagnosis or a surgical procedure requires nursing care. A nurse reviews the clinically relevant data and, with the patient, develops an individualized plan of care articulating specific individualized care for that patient based on the Nursing Process. This model includes medical and nursing orders with the EHR system. The nurse documents the nursing related content for a specific PPOC using coded nursing terminology.
2. The PPOC is stored within an HIT system.
3. During the inpatient stay, the nurse continually evaluates actions and reviews the PPOC frequently to ensure quality care is maintained. The PPOC is revised as needed. For example: availability of new information or a change in the patient's condition. (IHE, 2011, p. 14)

Plan of Care Steps for the Transfer of Care Context

1. When a patient is transferred to another facility the PPOC is reviewed and updated as needed to promote continuity of care.
2. The updated PPOC is exchanged with the destination facility.
3. The PPOC is reviewed at the destination facility and updated as needed. (IHE, 2011, p. 14)

Project Implementation

The current data element layout of the 40-paper nursing assessment documents was replicated in HTML and coded for display on a web page using JavaScript. The content components of the World Wide Web Consortium (W3C) were used to create the PPOC using the structured, standardized, coded CCC nursing terminology concepts that *a priori* supported the nursing workflow and evidence-based practice at Bumrungrad International Hospital. In the HTML layout, MEDCIN findings for documented patient signs and symptoms automatically presented relevant CCC concepts within the Nursing Process format. This process carried a CCC code to the PPOC based on a coded MEDCIN finding that allows for the aggregation of nursing data for future nursing research and analysis. The CCC System information model guided the integration of nursing data in the PPOC and optimized continuity using the Nursing Process. The HTML PPOC layouts using MEDCIN and CCC demonstrated data continuity between the nursing assessments of patient signs and symptoms and individualized plans of care. The PPOC enabled the reuse of patient data to offer new insight into the complexity of care performed by nurses.

The NI team envisioned implementing the PPOC on 10-inch wireless tablets to expand at-the-bedside patient care as well as facilitate safety in the hand-off of patient care communication. Initial attention focused on the capacity of the wireless network. A systematic assessment of wireless capacity was conducted prior to implementation to prepare any mitigation strategies for changes to nursing workflow caused by wireless response time. This assessment served to avoid a common pitfall of unexpected insufficient device connectivity. Further, the NI team exercised due diligence in calculating for, and ensuring, the availability of a sufficient number of devices for documentation. The NI team also involved several hospital committees (nursing, physician, and medical records) in planning efforts for the development of new hospital policies for electronic documentation involving, for example, interward patient connections (transfers and admissions), automated signature attributions, and care documentation addendums.

Staff training took place from September to November 2013 with an initial 90-minute review of the ANA Nursing Process and the CCC. *Super-user* nurses received 2-hour hands-on training, including how to use the tablet and how the Nursing Process was integrated during the nursing assessments, care planning, and progress note documentation. The NI team organized and conducted 148 training classes for 305 nurses (21 hours of training per person) to be "ready" to use the system and evaluated each individual nurse on their acquired skills before being authorized to access the electronic system (Figures 5.4 and 5.5). The NI team also organized training classes for 241

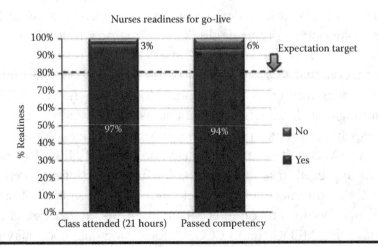

Figure 5.4   Bumrungrad nurse readiness for "go-live."

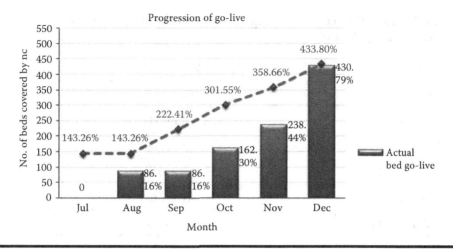

Figure 5.5   Bumrungrad ward progression of implementation for "go-live."

nurses (12 classes) on "how to access nursing intervention information of the patients whose information was electronically documented." The NI team also confirmed through surveys that the electronic nursing documentation was meeting nurses' needs and resolving any training needs to ensure the consistent compliance of practice with nursing policies and procedures.

With the first parallel application testing scheduled in 4 weeks, the NI team and selected super-users checked the electronic assessment documentation and care plan processes, focusing on how the information system and equipment worked together to support innovative patient care. The NI team and super-users assisted with the final stages of building assessment layouts and validated the information linkages for "abnormal" findings (e.g., coughing, disorientation) to CCC Nursing Diagnoses, Goals, Nursing Interventions, and Intervention actions.

In February 2014, the PPOC project launched in 14 beds on a 50-bed medical-surgical ward with 26 nurses participating. A majority of nurses on the selected ward surveyed had "self-identified" as early technology adopters (Rogers, 1962). There was strong nursing leadership support on the selected ward expressed for the project. There were two phases of implementation:

■ Phase 1 from February to March 2014 involved 75 patients.
■ Phase 2 from May to July 2014 involved 82 patients.

During Phase 1 and Phase 2, the NI team simultaneously conducted timed, parallel observations between paper forms and electronic documentation, focusing on the ability of the PPOC to support patient assessments

Table 5.3   Electronic Nursing Documentation Implementation "Go-Live" by Ward

Department	2014 Nursing Ward "Go-Live" Dates
Ward 6	21 October
Ward 7A	20 August
Ward 8A	15 December
Ward 8CD	15 December
Ward 9A	13 November
Ward 9CD	25 November
Ward 10A	15 December
Ward 10CD	15 December
Ward 11A	25 August
Ward 11C	5 August
Ward 11D	14 August
Ward 12A	15 October
Ward 12CD	15 December

and care plan documentation. Of 50 nursing assessment layouts created in HTML, 18 layouts were selected for phased implementation. (*Note*: In each phase, paper and electronic assessments were reviewed for completeness concurrently and in parallel for each patient to avoid any loss of data integrity or effect on patient care.) (Table 5.3)

Results

The initial plan for project implementation was to expand the use of the electronic nursing documentation system to additional wards when the nurses of those wards requested and preferred electronic documentation. The PPOC profile, using structured, coded CCC nursing terminology for patient care, was implemented in August 2014. By December 2014, project expansion covered 430 inpatient beds (79% of all available inpatient beds). Currently, the PPOC has been used to prompt individualized PPOCs for 1755 new admissions, or 41% of all new admissions. The PPOC is hospital wide,

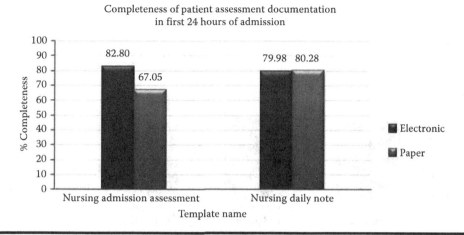

Figure 5.6   **Medical record completeness of documentation.**

with MEDCIN and CCC for 97% of new inpatient admission assessment documentation.

A descriptive analysis of the concurrent phased documentation reviews found electronic documentation replaced subjective nursing descriptions and provided a cohesive and objective picture of a patient's overall condition. In each phase, the PPOC successfully carried the appropriate CCC codes from the nursing assessment to the nursing plan of care. A retrospective review of the first 24 hours of admission documentation found the completeness of nursing assessments was higher than the former method of data format conversion and document storage in the CPOE system compared with average 2013 scores. In Phase 2, documentation completeness was higher than in Phase 1. The review found there was no data loss in either trial phase (Figure 5.6).

A user satisfaction survey during the trial period showed that overall nursing satisfaction in Phase 2 was higher (2.91%) than in Phase 1 (2.72%), and the nurses agreed to use the electronic documentation system instead of written (paper) documentation (Figure 5.7). A random comparison of electronic documentation completeness during the first 24 hours after admission compared with paper documentation completeness from September to December is shown in Figure 5.8.

Lessons Learned

The partnership of nursing and technology is vital for designing nursing practice environments for the exchange and interoperability of nursing

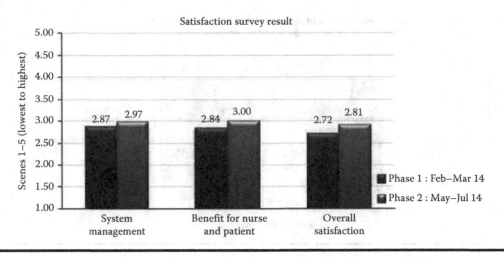

Figure 5.7   Bumrungrad electronic documentation satisfaction.

data, and PPOC content structures facilitate the provision of patient-centric care for the entire healthcare team. Nursing care plans are used to foster the comparability of nursing data and information across patient populations and support a continuous, efficient, shared clinical understanding of a patient's care history. Keenan et al. (2006) note simultaneous access to patients' histories by the healthcare team aids interdisciplinary communication and decision-making about the future care of patients. Nursing plans of care are a common language. When the primary function of nursing documentation is to communicate professional nursing

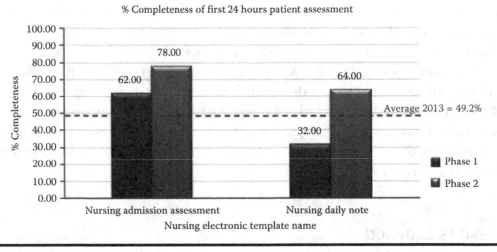

Figure 5.8   Electronic nursing documentation completion (medical record review of 833 discharged patients: 677 written [paper] documents and 156 electronic documents).

assessments about patients to other nurses and providers and ensure the visibility of continuity of care, the PPOC is an important technology resource asset.

There were significant changes that made Phase 2 documentation more complete than that of Phase 1 and resulted in higher satisfaction toward electronic documentation.

1. Nursing care plans were harmonized with standard physician treatment plans.
2. Integrated automated electronic record system dates and times for compliance with the medical records system.
3. The development of an automated monitoring and reporting system for documentation compliance.
4. Improved Wi-Fi signals that covered most of the nursing work areas.
5. The development of an *auto-signature* system.

Other lessons learned from the PPOC implementation project are as follows:
1. Engage nurses in every step of system development.
2. Use the following PPOC content configuration:
   a. Achieve integrated patient assessments and nursing plans of care.
   b. Require a specific nursing diagnosis, goal, intervention, and outcome for each patient.
   c. Use an integrated documentation plan of care.
   d. System configurations should use familiar data structures and ANA frameworks.
3. HTML configuration accelerates functional and operational development.
4. Incremental expansion of electronic implementation based on ward-assessed readiness is successful in reaching 100% adoption with nursing governance.
5. Plan to increase electronic assessment paper conversions to 12 layouts per year.
6. Plan review and update schedules for care plan linkages to evidence-based practice.
7. Offer feedback to SDOs on obstacles in the practical application of standards in the designing of electronic nursing care documentation.
8. Support staff potential and system competency.

As the world moves toward the global sharing of health information, nurses are able to exchange data through the use of the PPOC profile and use nursing concepts to synthesize data to improve patient care. Gordon (2005) notes that documentation may be the most critical factor in a patient's treatment and recovery. Understanding the health impact of nursing care on patient outcomes may be the key to improving quality in healthcare systems. In 2010, Thede reflected, "Two significant challenges have always faced nursing: (1) how to differentiate nursing's contributions to patient care from those of medicine; and (2) how to incorporate descriptions of nursing care into the health record in a manner that is commensurate with its importance to patients' welfare." The PPOC reduces healthcare fragmentation and expands the interoperability of data for optimal patient care through the effective coordination of care, which will solve the largest global gap in health information—care data collected and recorded by nurses!

References

American Academy of Family Physicians. (2015). Coordination of care. Retrieved from http://www.aafp.org/about/policies/all/definition-care.html.

American Nurses Association. (2010). *Nursing: Scope and Standards of Practice*, 2nd edition. Silver Spring, MD: Nursingbooks.org.

American Recovery and Reinvestment Act of 2009 (ARRA). (2009). PL 111-5. Washington, DC: Federal Register.

ANA. (2012). The value of nursing care coordination: A white paper of the American nurses association. Retrieved from http://www.nursingworld.org/carecoordinationwhitepaper.

ANA. (2015a). What is nursing? Retrieved from http://www.nursingworld.org/EspeciallyForYou/What-is-Nursing.

ANA (2015b). Nursing Process. Retrieved from http://www.nursingworld.org/especiallyforyou/studentnurses/thenursingprocess.aspx.

ANA. (2016). Care coordination and registered nurses' essential role. Retrieved from http://nursingworld.org/MainMenuCategories/Policy-Advocacy/Positions-and-Resolutions/ANAPositionStatements/Position-Statements-Alphabetically/Care-Coordination-and-Registered-Nurses-Essential-Role.htm.

Atherly, A., and Thorpe, K.E. (2011). Analysis of the treatment effect of Healthway's Medicare Health Support Phase 1 pilot on Medicare costs. *Population Health Management*, 14(1), 23–28.

Bumrungrad International. (2015). About us. Retrieved from https://www.bumrungrad.com/en/about-us/overview.

Burns, M., Dyer, M.B., and Bailit, M. (2014). Reducing overuse and misuse: State strategies to improve quality and cost of health care. Robert Wood Johnson Foundation. Retrieved from http://www.ohsu.edu/xd/research/centers-institutes/evidence-based-policy-center/upload/Bailit__Reducing-Overuse-and-Misuse-State-strategies-to-improve-quality.pdf.

Chalmers, R.J.G. (2006). Health care terminology for the electronic era. *Mayo Clinic Proc*; 81, 619–624.

Clinical Care Classification System. (n.d.). Retrieved from https://en.wikipedia.org/wiki/Clinical_Care_Classification_System.

Ebright, P.R. (2010). The complex work of RNs: Implications for healthy work environments. *Online Journal of Nursing*. Retrieved from http://www.nursingworld.org/MainMenuCategories/ANAMarketplace/ANAPeriodicals/OJIN/TableofContents/Vol152010/No1Jan2010/Complex-Work-of-RNs.html.

Endsley, M.R. (1995). Toward a theory of situation awareness in dynamic systems. *Human Factors*; 37, 32–64.

FHIM. (n.d.). Care plan. Retrieved from http://www.fhims.org/content/_DV.q1IAY0E.eG.z0.d.k.a.dE.l.r.kQ-content.html.

Goltra, P.S. (1978). *MEDCIN®: A New Nomenclature for Clinical Medicine*. New York: Springer.

Gordon, S. (2005). *Nursing against the Odds: How Healthcare Cost Cutting, Media Stereotypes, and Medical Hubris Undermine Nurses and Patient Care*. New York: Cornell University Press.

Hardiker, N.R., Bakken, S., Casey, A., and Hoy, D. (2002). Formal nursing terminology systems: Means to an end. *Journal of Biomedical Informatics*; 35, 298–305.

HHS. Strategic goal 1: Strengthen health care. Retrieved from http://www.hhs.gov/about/strategic-plan/strategic-goal-1/index.html#obj_b.

HHS. (2008). Office of the National Coordinator for Health Information Technology (ONC), DHHS. Notice of availability: Secretarial recognition of certain Healthcare Information Technology Standards Panel (HITSP) interoperability specifications and the standards they contain as interoperability standards for health information technology. Federal Register: vol. 73, January 23, p. 3973.

HITSP. (2009a). HITSP biosurveillance interoperability specifications; IS02, version 2.1. Retrieved from http://www.hitsp.org/ConstructSet_Details.aspx?&PrefixAlpha=1&PrefixNumeric=02.

HITSP. (2009b). HITSP background. Retrieved from http://www.hitsp.org/background.aspx.

IHE International. (2009). IHE PCC technical framework supplement: Patient plan of care (PPOC), PPOC Rev. 1.0, 2009-05-2901.

IHE International. (2011). IHE patient care coordination (PCC) technical framework supplement: Patient plan of care (PPOC), trial implementation.

IHE International Wiki. (2014). Integrating the Healthcare Enterprise. Retrieved from http://wiki.ihe.net/index.php?title=Main_Page.

IHE International Wiki. (2016). Profiles. Retrieved from http://wiki.ihe.net/index.php?title=Profiles.

Integrating the Healthcare Enterprise, International (IHE). (2008). Coded Nursing Documentation (CND; CDOC-NT). Retrieved from http://webcache.google-usercontent.com/search?q=cache:JayqoP-FwDcJ:wiki.ihe.net/images/8/8c/Detailed_Proposal_Coded_Nursing_Documentation_Profile_Oct22_2008.doc+&cd=2&hl=en&ct=clnk&gl=us.

International Organization for Standardization. (2010). *Mapping of Terminologies to Classifications: DTR 123000*. Geneva, Switzerland: ISO Press.

IOM. (2001). *Crossing the Quality Chasm: A New Health System for the 21st Century.* Washington, DC: National Academies Press.

IOM. (2011). *The Healthcare Imperative: Lowering Costs and Improving Outcomes; Workshop Series Summary.* Washington, DC: The National Academies Press. Retrieved from http://iom.nationalacademies.org/Reports/2011/The-Healthcare-Imperative Lowering-Costs-and-Improving-Outcomes.aspx#sthash.EbOgB53f.dpuf.

Keenan, G.M., Yakel, E., and Marriott, D. (2006) HANDS: A revitalized technology supported care planning method to improve nursing handoffs. Paper presented at the 9th International Congress on Nursing Informatics, June 2006, Seoul, Korea.

Kozier, B., Erb, G., Berman, A., and Snyder, S. (2004). *Fundamentals of Nursing: Constructs, Process, and Practice*, 2nd edition. Upper Saddle River, NJ: Pearson/Prentice Hall.

Marek, K., Adams, S., Stetzer, F., Popejoy, L., and Rantz, M. (2010). The relationship of community based nurse care coordination to costs in the Medicare and Medicaid programs. *Research in Nursing and Health*; 33, 235–242.

ONC. (2015a). Benefits of electronic health records (EHRs). Retrieved from http://healthit.gov/providers-professionals/benefits-electronic-health-records-ehrs.

ONC. (2015b). Benefits of EHRs: Health care quality and convenience. Retrieved from http://www.healthit.gov/providers-professionals/health-care-quality-convenience.

Orszag, P. R. (2008). The overuse, underuse, and misuse of health care. Testimony before the Senate Committee on Finance. 110th Congress. Retrieved from http://www.cbo.gov/sites/default/files/cbofiles/ftpdocs/95xx/doc9567/07-17-healthcare_testimony.pdf.

Owens, M.K. (2011). Inefficiently delivered services, costs of uncoordinated care, Chapter 3, pp. 131–138 in IOM (2011), *The Healthcare Imperative: Lowering Costs and Improving Outcomes; Workshop Series Summary*, Washington, DC: The National Academies Press.

Richesson, R.L., and Krischer, J. (2007). Data standards in clinical research: Gaps, overlaps, challenges and future directions. *Journal of the American Medical Informatics Association*; 14(6): 687–696.

Rogers, E.M. (1962). *Diffusion of Innovations.* New York: The Free Press.

Saba, V.K. (1992). The classification of home health care nursing diagnoses and interventions. *Caring*; 10(3), 50–57.

Saba, V.K. (2007). *Clinical Care Classification (CCC) System Manual: A Guide to Nursing Documentation.* New York: Springer.

Saba, V.K. (2012). *Clinical Care Classification (CCC) System: Version 2.5*, 2nd edition. New York: Springer.

Saba, V.K., and Whittenburg, L. (2008) Coded Nursing Documentation (CND; CDOC-NT). Retrieved from http://wiki.ihe.net/images/8/8c/Detailed_Proposal_Coded_Nursing_Documentation_Profile_Oct22_2008.doc.

Schlossman, D.M. (2013). Continuity of care in the United States. Retrieved from http://www.himss.org/News/NewsDetail.aspx?ItemNumber=22261.

S&I. (2012). Longitudinal Coordination of Care work group: A community led initiative, care plan terms & proposed definitions, December 2012. Retrieved from http://wiki.siframework.org/LCC+Longitudinal+Care+Plan+%28LCP%29+SWG.

S&I. (2013). Longitudinal Coordination of Care interoperable care plan exchange use case v2.0. Retrieved from http://wiki.hl7.org/images/c/c4/LCC_Care_Plan_Exchange_Use_Case_FINAL.pdf.

S&I. (2015). Retrieved from http://wiki.siframework.org/Home.

Thede, L.Q., and Sewell, J.P. (2010). *Informatics and Nursing: Opportunities and Challenges*, 3rd edition. Philadelphia, PA: Lippincott, Williams & Wilkins.

Whittenburg, L. (ed.). (2013). *Health Information and Management Systems Society (HIMSS) Dictionary of Healthcare Information Technology Terms, Acronyms and Organizations*, 3rd edition. Chicago, IL: HIMSS.

Chapter 6

Diagnostic Imaging at eHealth Ontario

Laura Bright, Angela Lianos, and Sue Schneider

Contents

Background

The Ontario healthcare sector is a very complex environment, where tens of thousands of healthcare providers of different types work within a diverse set of public healthcare institutions, such as hospitals, rehabilitation centers, continuing care, mental health services, long-term care facilities, and community health agencies, as well as private sector enterprises providing supplementary care such as dental care, pharmacies, and laboratories. The healthcare system is governed by a province of Ontario government portfolio, the Ministry of Health and Long-Term Care (MOHLTC). Healthcare is a large component of the Ontario government's budget, with healthcare spending at over $80 billion and 11.3% of GDP in 2014 (Canadian Institute for Health Information 2014), and as factors such as population growth, aging populations, and increased rates of chronic and complex diseases are increasingly prevalent, these costs only continue to grow. Although the province is responsible for a large portion of the funding for healthcare in Ontario, there are other sources of funding the provinces and territories depend on in the form of payments from the Canadian or federal government based on an action plan with billions of dollars to support shared goals across the country under the Canada Health Accord, in renegotiation starting in early 2016 (Canadian Press 2015), with negotiations completed for most provinces and territories by March 2017 (Government of Canada 2017). Canada Health Infoway is also a source of investment in digital health in Canada, and has been coinvesting in local, regional, provincial, and territorial projects across Canada since 2001, including the eHealth Ontario Diagnostic Imaging Common Service (DI CS) initiative (Canada Health Infoway 2016).

The provincial government established eHealth Ontario in September 2008 as an independent agency of the Ontario MOHLTC, with the vision of creating a single, province-wide electronic health record (EHR) system. Achieving this goal requires a firm commitment to practical solutions, and this philosophy informs the agency's vision for digital healthcare. The favored approach is one that leverages the significant progress local and regional health service providers have made over the past decade in EHR system solutions designed to provide a longitudinal birth-to-death health record for every patient in the province.

The concept of the EHR, as opposed to the electronic medical record (EMR) software commonly used in hospitals and clinics, refers to a system or integrated network of systems that combines all of the health-related information about a patient into a single, unified view. In particular, when we talk about the provincial EHR for Ontario, we are talking about a set of clinical data repositories along with a number of registries holding nonclinical data and an associated integration layer called the *health information access layer* (HIAL) that provides services for point-of-service systems to use the data contained in the EHR.

The province's 155 (Ontario MOHLTC n.d.) hospital systems have widely adopted electronic recordkeeping and, as of 2015, more than 11,650 community-based clinicians (Ontario MD 2015) representing approximately 9 million Ontarians have or are in the process of implementing single-organization EMR software solutions in their practices. The province also has 14 regional health organizations, called *local health integration networks* (LHINs), that have a mandate to plan, fund, and provide integration services for all of the providers and provider organizations in the province. Many of these hospitals and clinicians, along with the LHINs, have been working together to integrate local solutions into regional integration hubs (eHealth Ontario 2015). If the agency is to achieve the goal of establishing a single health record for each Ontario resident in a cost-effective manner, leveraging the best of the regional integration hubs must be a key part of the overall strategy.

The implementation of a provincial EHR is expected to have a number of benefits (eHealth Ontario 2015), including

- Improved care through timely, secure, accurate, and complete information
- Improved safety and reduced potential for adverse effects
- Improved security of confidential health information
- Improved practice efficiencies and reduced health system costs

eHealth Ontario developed Ontario's eHealth Blueprint (eHealth Ontario 2014) aligned with the Canada Health Infoway Electronic Health Record Solution (EHRS) Blueprint (Canada Health Infoway n.d.), a technology framework for enabling the sharing of patient health information across health service providers, to guide the vision and direction for how health information technology is used by information systems to interoperate. Building on the vision and direction from the blueprint and extensive consultation with the MOHLTC and stakeholders, including clinicians, Ontario's EHR Connectivity Strategy (eHealth Ontario 2008–2016) has been developed to inform investment and integration decisions. This strategic connectivity guidance includes an asset inventory and identifies provincial assets to be used with local and regional information technology solutions as part of Ontario's EHR. The MOHLTC provides the strategic direction for the health system in Ontario, including electronic health, and funds eHealth Ontario in this important transition to the future state of Ontario's EHR. In addition to work with Canada Health Infoway for architecture and standards alignment, and specific investment projects used to advance digital health in Canada, eHealth Ontario works closely with the MOHLTC and many contracted regional and local partners to advance the implementation and adoption of Ontario's EHR. One specific project of interest to standardization and integration comes from eHealth Ontario's diagnostic imaging (DI) program, and is part of the agency's overall strategy to improve patient care, safety, and access. By putting in place a stable technical infrastructure based on sound architecture and interoperable standards for DI, it guarantees that healthcare providers have access to vital clinical activity information systems when they need it. Now let's jump back to the early steps that set the stage for being able to achieve eHealth Ontario's DI CS, a complex multiyear initiative for eHealth Ontario.

In 2005, the Canada Health Infoway EHRS Blueprint was published, which outlined a separate DI service (Canada Health Infoway n.d.). Around that time, the MOHLTC eHealth Program issued a request for proposals (RFP) for the development of a province-wide DI strategy and options analysis to better integrate DI initiatives across Ontario for hospitals and independent health facilities (IHF), which are community-based nonhospital facilities that provide diagnostic services (ultrasound, x-ray, pulmonary function, nuclear medicine, and sleep studies) and/or surgical/treatment services (e.g., cataract surgery, dialysis, or plastic surgery). This strategy and options analysis was done by an external vendor, which resulted in some key strategy points that it was recommended eHealth Ontario adopt, including

- Support for potential projects and opportunities from regional stakeholders such as the Pan Northern Ontario Project (PNOP), the Toronto East Network (TEN), and the provincial Electronic Master Patient Index (EMPI)
- Development of DI archives as separate data assets

■ Decoupling of operational picture archive and communications systems (PACS) from diagnostic imaging repositories (DI-rs), sharing PACS where possible, establishing DI-rs, and expanding those to independent health facilities (IHF)

Over the next few years, as discussions with hospitals and funders ensued, six projects were created that ultimately resulted in the creation of four DI-rs, roughly corresponding to four geographic catchment areas in the province. All organizations in these catchment areas that perform DI services would populate the DI-r for their area with all images and results from their organization, with the result that any hospital-based clinician with access to the DI-r would have access to all of the imaging studies pertaining to their patient that had been performed in the area, without having to query every site. The four DI-rs are

■ Southwestern Ontario Diagnostic Imaging Network (SWODIN), comprised of 70 hospital sites and 6 IHF hubs in LHINs 1–4
■ Greater Toronto Area (GTA) West DI-r, comprised of 33 hospital sites and 2 IHF hubs in LHINs 5, 6, part of 7, part of 8, and 12
■ Hospital Diagnostic Imaging Repository Services (HDIRS), comprised of 38 hospital sites and 9 IHF hubs in part of LHIN 7, part of LHIN 8, and LHINs 9–10
■ Northern and Eastern Diagnostic Imaging Network (NEODIN), comprised of 67 hospital sites and 7 IHF hubs in LHINs 11, 13, and 14

Several of the projects that were identified in the original strategy and options analysis were also incorporated into these four DI-rs, including the PNOP, which ended up as part of NEODIN, and the TEN projects, which ended up as part of HDIRS.

As an example of how DI-rs would be used to benefit patients, consider a case where a patient visits a hospital in one area and in the future goes to another hospital in that region because he or she has been referred for more specialized care. The specialist can utilize that repository's viewer to retrieve a list of all the diagnostic exams that patient has received in the region to inform better decision-making. For example, in the SWODIN area, there was a boy who was transferred from one of the smaller hospitals to the London Health Sciences Centre. The technologist scanning him was able to see his prior exam information utilizing the SWODIN DI-r and, as a result, performed a different scan on him than she would have had she not seen the previous results and identified an issue that would have gone undetected.

As a result of the DI-r making prior imaging available, the clinician is able to treat the patient without the interruption in their workflow that sending out a request for these results would cause, and the patient spends less time waiting for care. The time to reach diagnosis is reduced and there is a reduction in unnecessary duplicate exams, along with a corresponding reduction in unnecessary radiation exposure for the patient. There is work in progress to provide more quantitative data and metrics on the benefits of DI-rs; however, preliminary studies show unnecessary exams have been avoided.

Current Status of DI-rs and the Concept of DI CS

As of September 2013, the DI-r projects had progressed to the extent that all hospitals in Ontario that performed DI exams were integrated with one of the four regional repositories based on their geography, and by March 2015, 3.4 million exams from digitally enabled IHFs were integrated into one of the four regional repositories. Throughout the fiscal year 2014–2015, over 12 million exams were stored in the four DI-rs, and the DI-rs currently house over 62 million exams.

While there were significant clinical benefits derived from the implementation and integration of the DI-rs, the requirement to make all diagnostic information available to all healthcare settings in the province still existed. There were three main components to this requirement:

1. The four DI-rs were self-contained. DI results could only be accessed within the regional repository where the diagnostic exam originated, but there was clinical demand for cross-regional sharing.
2. Access to DI-rs was not enabled for community-based healthcare providers, outside of hospitals and IHFs, where the majority of care occurs. There was clinical demand for access to DI-rs from referring physicians, general practitioners, and specialists in community-based settings, and ~20,000 physicians did not have immediate online access to current and prior DI information to assist them in making timely treatment decisions.
3. Many IHFs crossed regional boundaries and required access to images from multiple DI-rs.

As a result of these requirements, the DI CS initiative was established to address provincial sharing. This initiative is intended to enable and support the sharing and viewing of diagnostic reports and images across Ontario to all hospital- and community-based providers anywhere, at any time, using the tools best suited to their work practice. Figure 6.1 represents the vision of the DI CS initiative.

As an example of how DI CS is used and how it impacts patient care, a clinician can now extract a provincial longitudinal view of a patient's diagnostic exams. For example, there was a patient in North Bay (part of the NEODIN DI-r) who was having cancer surgery in Toronto. The oncologist in Toronto pulled up her report from DI CS and adjusted her course of care: what was going to be a much more complicated treatment was reduced in its complexity and severity based on the information the oncologist was able to see, and she was on a plane back to North Bay within three days (Figure 6.2).

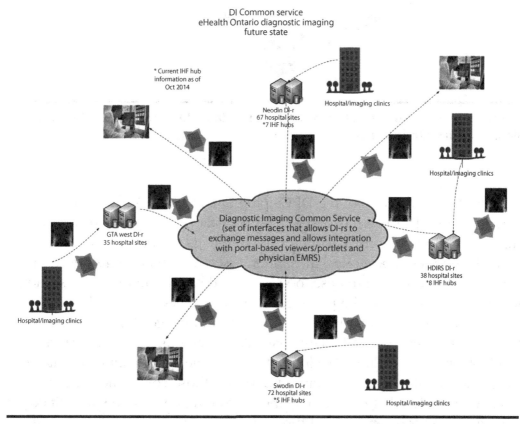

Figure 6.1   Diagnostic Imaging Common Service. (From © eHealth Ontario 2015, reprinted with permission, eHealth Ontario 2017.)

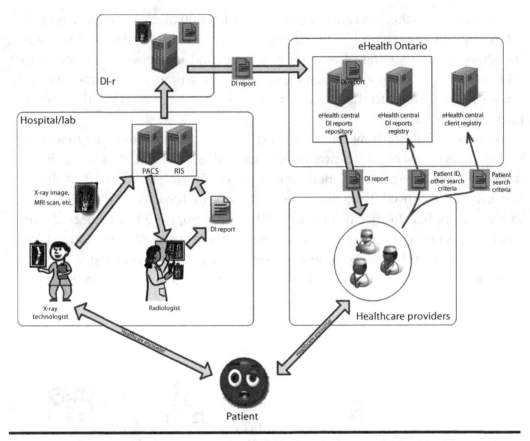

Figure 6.2 DI CS workflow. (From © eHealth Ontario 2015, reprinted with permission, eHealth Ontario 2017.)

With the introduction of the DI CS program, eHealth Ontario is coordinating the four DI-r projects covering all hospitals in Ontario and providing funding support and provincial infrastructure (e.g., the provincial network in addition to the repositories, integration assets, and other registries leveraged for DI CS). These are described in more detail in the following section to give providers across the province access to the system and allow for the cross-regional sharing of patients' reports and images from any location across the province. The DI-rs have data center and staffing costs as a result of running the DI-r. eHealth Ontario and the participating hospitals of the particular DI-r provide funding support for those costs. There are different cost models, but eHealth Ontario is working on a more streamlined approach to address operational funding.

eHealth Ontario Technical Environment

A key component of the overall eHealth Ontario strategy is Ontario's eHealth Blueprint (eHealth Ontario 2014). Providing a firm definition of the future state of the EHR for Ontario, the blueprint defines the elements required to realize the agency's goals for the EHR and describes the architectural principles and patterns that will be employed to deliver it. Encompassing and built on eHealth Ontario's foundational principles of privacy, collaborative governance, and the adoption of standards, the blueprint specifies the many roles and responsibilities of stakeholders throughout the healthcare sector (eHealth Ontario 2014). It provides the guidance needed for those stakeholders to innovate locally through their regional hubs while continuing to align with eHealth Ontario's overall strategy.

The blueprint provides multiple views:

■ The business view (Figure 6.3), which represents eHealth Ontario's view of the healthcare sector in Ontario, including the business-level services that the agency provides, its stakeholders, business objectives, and capabilities.
■ The information view (Figure 6.4), which provides a model of the information contained in the EHR in Ontario and provides a structure for managing health information from multiple sources.
■ The systems view (Figure 6.5), which describes the systems and applications in the core infrastructure required to build the Ontario EHR.

In order to achieve the full potential of the EHR and maximize the clinical value, it is important that all of the systems comprising the EHR, including the DI CS infrastructure, align with all three layers of the blueprint.

Key Architecture Components

Client Registry

One of the central challenges in every healthcare interoperability project is the unambiguous identification of the patient, and there are many processes and solutions to making sure that the information being exchanged all belongs to the correct patient. In Ontario, every person who receives care, regardless of their eligibility for government-funded health services, is

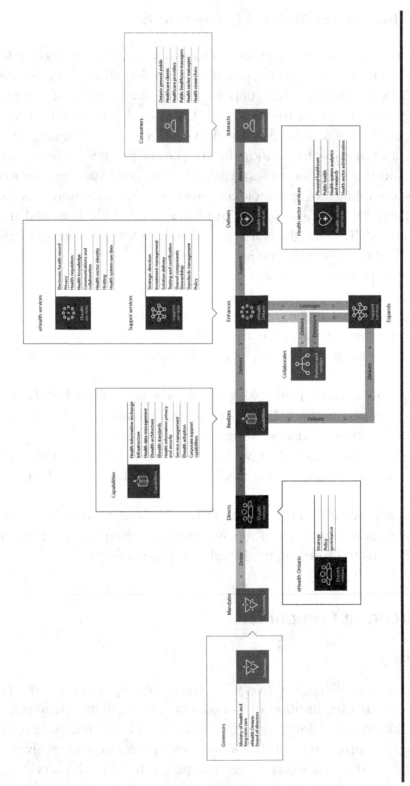

Figure 6.3   eHealth Ontario architecture business view. (From © eHealth Ontario 2014, reprinted with permission, eHealth Ontario 2017.)

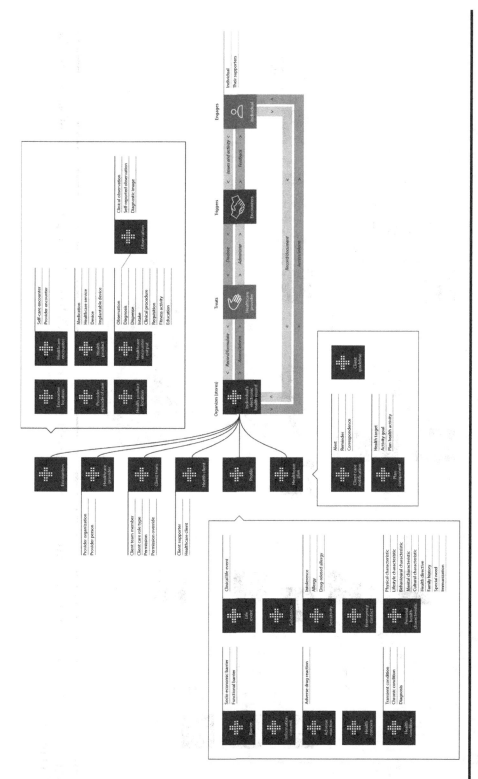

Figure 6.4 eHealth Ontario architecture information view. (From © eHealth Ontario 2014, reprinted with permission, eHealth Ontario 2017.)

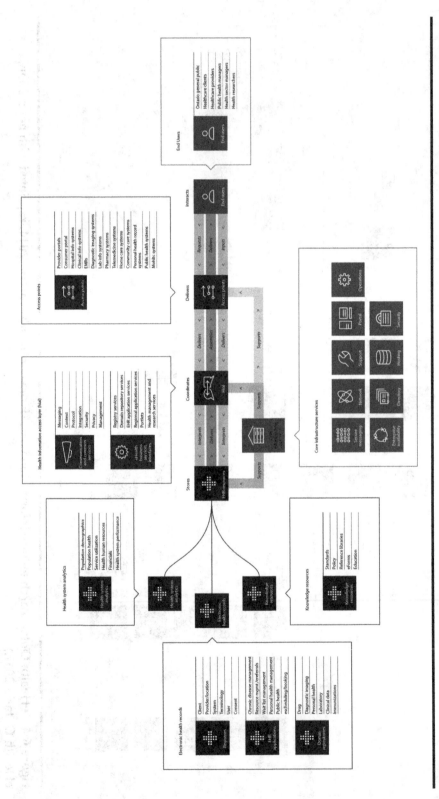

Figure 6.5   eHealth Ontario architecture systems view. (From © eHealth Ontario 2014, reprinted with permission, eHealth Ontario 2017.)

regarded as a healthcare client and is assigned a unique identifier, used uniformly across the province. The Client Registry is the definitive source for a healthcare client's identity, facilitating the unique, accurate, and reliable identification of individual clients and others who receive care in Ontario, across the disciplines in the healthcare sector. The registry contains demographic and identification data for healthcare clients registered in one or more facilities with which eHealth Ontario is sharing information, as well as a service that matches records from different sources belonging to a single healthcare client. For example, someone may have been treated in several hospitals; each hospital has an electronic record of the patient's interactions with that hospital, but each hospital system uses a unique identification number. It is important that the provincial EHR be able to recognize that these records all actually refer to the same individual (eHealth Ontario 2008–2016).

Examples of services provided by the registry include

- Validating healthcare client identity information
- Searching and resolving information from multiple sources that refer to the same healthcare client identity
- Obtaining summary and detailed demographic information about a healthcare client
- Adding and updating a healthcare client record
- Merging and unmerging healthcare client records (because they either do or do not refer to the same individual)
- Reconciling duplicates
- Managing publish/subscribe notifications of adds, updates, merges, and splits to downstream systems (eHealth Ontario 2008–2016)

Provider Registry

The Provider Registry is the authoritative source of information about providers and healthcare service delivery locations for use by all EHR solutions. It facilitates the unique and accurate identification of any individual or organization that provides health services in Ontario, or who participates in the collection, use, or disclosure of protected health information (PHI) across the continuum of care. The registry assigns a unique provincial identifier to each provider and maintains information about them, including professional accreditations (e.g., licenses, professions, specialties). It is fed by regulatory colleges, MOHLTC databases, hospitals, and other organizations (eHealth Ontario 2008–2016).

The Provider Registry is designed to address the business need to

▪ Positively identify providers
▪ Retrieve information on providers, including credentials, status, documented restrictions of activity, work locations, and relevant healthcare organization affiliations and local privileges
▪ Search and resolve a provider's identity
▪ Search and retrieve provider organization data and locations
▪ Obtain provider information (e.g., current status of professional accreditations) (eHealth Ontario 2008–2016)

Health Information Access Layer

At the core of Ontario's eHealth Blueprint and tying all of these infrastructure pieces together is the HIAL. The HIAL is the central messaging application for the EHR, based on an enterprise service bus (ESB) and acting as the central transaction coordinator for all services that are a part of the EHR. Each transaction that goes through the EHR goes through several steps and requires multiple services to be processed, including authentication, terminology translation, and the application of consent rules, among others. The HIAL has awareness of all of these transactions, as well as the series of steps each has to take, and coordinates the execution of these steps from service request to final response. The core business and data processing logic associated with a clinical domain is expected to be handled and processed by the line-of-business application itself, once the HIAL passes the appropriately formed service request to it (eHealth Ontario 2008–2016).

The HIAL's fundamental capabilities and duties include the following:

▪ Recognizing and having awareness of all transactions handled by the HIAL
▪ Coordinating the execution of all EHR transactions from start (service request) to finish (service response sent to requester)
▪ Monitoring and managing the state of all EHR transactions
▪ Monitoring, controlling, and routing message exchanges between services
▪ Resolving and managing contention between communicating service components
▪ Controlling the deployment and versioning of services

■ Providing commonly needed transaction processing services, including event handling and event choreography

■ Data transformation and mapping, message and event queuing and sequencing, security, error/exception handling, message parsing and validation, protocol conversion, enforcing the proper quality of communication services

■ Providing commonly needed and commoditized EHR business services, including validation of the asserted authentication of the end user involved with a transaction, role-based service access, authorization of the end user involved with a transaction, application of coarse-grained consent directives for disclosure of information

■ Validation and resolution of key enterprise reference identifiers for transactions, including client, provider, and provider organization involved in clinical transactions

■ Catering for the optional application of business logic rules associated with specific business domains (eHealth Ontario 2008–2016)

Figure 6.6 illustrates the logical architecture for the HIAL in relation to the registry and repository for DI CS.

Consent Registry

The Consent Registry provides a central location for the storage of a patient's instructions as to who can access their records and in what circumstances. These instructions are called *consent directives*. The provincial consent management solution enables the uniform enforcement of a patient's privacy directives for all EHR transactions. If a patient issues a consent directive blocking a specific provider's access to their information, the Consent Registry ensures that directive will be enforced at all times.

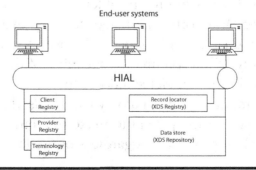

Figure 6.6   HIAL logical architecture.

The Consent Registry is integrated with the HIAL, so patient consent directives are applied to all provincial EHR transactions going into DI CS (eHealth Ontario 2008–2016).

Terminology Registry

Healthcare systems may use different local names, codes, or wording for the same clinical concepts. As an example, when a clinician wants to record that a patient had a heart attack, they may say "heart attack" or "myocardial infarction" or abbreviate it as "MI." These terms all mean the same thing but would not be interpreted to be the same by a computer. When health-care data from different sources are being shared, it is essential to be able to translate or resolve these differences, to ensure correct interpretation by both people and systems.

This translation is done by using codes for the concepts being described, which translate human-readable names into names that can be interpreted by machines as well. These naming schemes are called *vocabularies* or *terminologies* and commonly originate and are governed by terminology authorities with editorial rules and licensing rights. Rules for mapping/translating from one set of terminology to another must be established and stored in accord with terminology best practices. Authoring and mapping tools will be used by terminology specialists to support the creation and maintenance of the terminology value sets and associations. The piece of infrastructure that stores these code sets and mappings and performs the translations between different codes is called the Terminology Registry.

The Terminology Registry is used as the "source of truth" for the SNOMED CT® codes that make up provincial terminology for DI CS. The DI CS provincial terminology is then mapped to the local hospital radiology information system (RIS) and PACS DI procedures to create a terminology map (e.g., local terms to provincial terms) for all hospitals or other organizations sending DI reports and images to the provincial DI CS. The Terminology Registry enables and supports the use of standard terminologies as a common way of interpreting the meaning of data in the images and reports from local to provincial solutions. In the case of DI CS, the DI procedure maps, modality, and anatomy can be used at the time of searching for DI studies for the patient to make the retrieval precise by presenting the provincial DI procedure regardless of the local naming (eHealth Ontario 2008–2016).

Overall Workflow

Consider a doctor at a hospital requesting the retrieval of a laboratory report from the EHR lab system. To fulfill the request, a number of steps have to be taken.

- The patient's identifier must be checked against the Client Registry, to retrieve the unique identifier for the patient from the local identifier.
- The provider's identifier must be checked against the Provider Registry to ensure they are a known provider.
- The provider's role must be checked against the security services to confirm they have permission to access the report.
- The report, patient, and provider must be checked against the Consent Registry to ensure the patient hasn't blocked access.
- The terminology service must be checked to translate any local codes used to those used by the HIAL.
- The report must be retrieved and returned to the provider's system.

Without a HIAL or other ESB system, this would require the hospital system to do a lot of complex coordination and to know a lot of details about the internal systems at the EHR. With the HIAL, that detail is hidden, and the integration with the end-user system is much simpler (eHealth Ontario 2008–2016).

Standards Development

An essential part of achieving interoperability and allowing components of the EHR to exchange information seamlessly and reliably is the appropriate selection and implementation of standards. For the EHR to work, everyone must agree on and use common processes, technology, data definitions, semantics, and formats for data exchange. The use of standards minimizes the cost of new implementations and allows new solutions and systems to participate in the EHR more easily. In the case of the DI CS initiative, it was important to include the capabilities of the four existing regional DI-rs, to minimize the amount of rework that had to be done on existing local information systems to liberate access to diagnostic studies. There were a number of considerations (Table 6.1) that made the solution decisions complex.

Table 6.1   Solution Considerations

Consideration	Scope
Existing vendor systems capabilities	• Differences in standards supported locally and regionally vs. provincially • Local hospitals/health facilities • Regional repositories • Provincial registry/repository
Data definitions	• Numerous local solutions • Four regional solutions • Provincial solution
Scaling for future expansion	• Inclusion of additional source systems • Foreign exam management
Terminology model	• Regional terminology registry • Provincial terminology services • Local terms data dictionaries (RIS and PACS) • Future HIS merging/unmerging of systems and mapping changes
Architectural approaches	• Alignment with HIAL and Ontario's eHealth Blueprint • Alignment to other provincial projects • Expectations for interoperability with other Ontario EHR systems
Source systems facilitating access to viewing	• Local and regional source systems to launch access to the provincial DI CS solution

In the early stages of the DI CS initiative, eHealth Ontario began a *conceptual standards assessment* and an environmental scan of standards in use in similar solutions to identify the potential standards available to support the business needs in Ontario for sharing DI reports and DI images. The environmental scan included looking at standards available to meet specific purposes as defined in the business requirements for the DI CS solution. Some of the standards assessed included Cross-Enterprise Document Sharing for Imaging (XDS-I) (Integrating the Healthcare Enterprise [IHE] 2008–2016) for the exchange of reports and image references, Health Level Seven International's Clinical Document Architecture (HL7 CDA R2) (HL7 2005) standards for representing the clinical content of the reports as documents, and SNOMED CT (SNOMED International 2016), a clinical terminology standard for code systems representing concepts for the procedures completed in DI study results.

eHealth Ontario also had a work in progress using the CDA (HL7 2005) standard, similar to the use by DI CS for another project in Ontario around the same time. This work involved the development of a CDA specification for a standardized document header. This work provided insights regarding the use of the HL7 CDA Release 2 (HL7 2005) standard used in the transmission of two specific documents from EMRs to a provincial registry for mother and baby health information, called the Better Outcomes Registry and Network (BORN 2016). This early opportunity provided experience with the CDA format and improved understanding of how to use the CDA header and metadata, and was valuable in increasing awareness of how CDA would work and what was involved in its implementation by the registry and the contributing EMRs. For consistency across the EHR, and ease of integration pathways for vendors and facilities that would be interacting with both DI CS and with the BORN project, it was important that the document format decisions made for DI CS be aligned with those in use for BORN. Keeping that alignment would allow other systems to consistently interpret documents from the EHR, regardless of the initiative that created them. As part of the solution design for DI CS, there were considerations that had to be assessed to ensure the needs for DI and future EHR solutions would be compatible. Table 6.1 provides insight into the considerations and the scope of factors considered.

Standards Governance Process

There were a number of working groups involved in the development of the DI CS standard. With a large project such as this, the standards guidance and implementation evolved over the course of the project, so backward compatibility for the standards in use in the four DI-rs and DI CS became important to ensure current and future interoperability.

The governance for the development of the standards for use in the DI CS project followed the structure and reporting requirements expected of all Canada Health Infoway investments. eHealth Ontario jointly funded the DI CS project with Canada Health Infoway and facilitated the alignment with Ontario's eHealth Blueprint (eHealth Ontario 2014) and other eHealth Ontario technical components. The governance structure for the working group tasked with the terminology standards work items included a working group with representation from the four DI-rs, Mohawk Shared Services (2016), eHealth Ontario, and Canada Health Infoway, as shown in Figure 6.7.

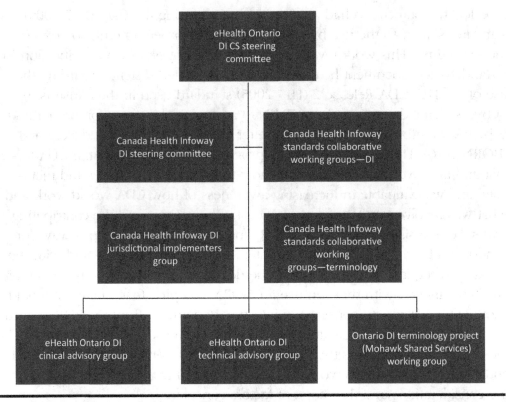

Figure 6.7   DI CS project: key governance structures. (From © eHealth Ontario 2015, reprinted with permission, eHealth Ontario 2017.)

Mohawk Shared Services, an organization that provides outsourced services to healthcare, played the role of delivery partner in the completion of the initial DI terminology set, terminology maps, and editorial guide, which it provided to eHealth Ontario for validation, ongoing maintenance, and sustained use with DI CS. Other sources of early consultation for the DI CS standard included Canada Health Infoway's Jurisdictional Implementation Group, where all Canadian provinces and territories with a DI project share and learn from each other, and the former Standards Collaborative working groups for DI and terminology, which were able to provide DI domain–specific business and technical insights and SNOMED CT–specific expertise (SNOMED International 2016), all of value to the development of the standard.

The approved DI CS standard was reviewed by representation from at least 24 key stakeholder organizations in Ontario and through eHealth Ontario's open standards review process. This robust, inclusive review builds consensus for the standard through a webinar introducing the standard and a process to submit comments. All in all, this outreach gives rise to implementable standards and important considerations from our stakeholders that otherwise would not be possible. In total, the standards review takes approximately 6 months from start to finish. Stakeholder engagement is a key component of our architecture and standards review processes at eHealth Ontario. The standards are developed or adapted during our project delivery governance, where the standards-specific content for the interoperability assessments are completed in alignment with the blueprint and the business requirements. All standards are jointly presented, in this case as DI and e-health standards, to bring the business and technical perspectives to the stakeholders in the EHR governance committees. This process supports an opportunity to hear from many stakeholders, and includes tracking for all comments and transparency of the status for comments that were included or will be considered for future inclusion in a standard. eHealth Ontario has an annual review process for work items being reviewed at the EHR governance committees and identifies any known changes to existing standards to determine if a full review, partial review, or informative update are required. As the DI CS standard continues to be implemented, there may be some minor changes required, so this maintenance approach makes this possible without a full review.

Developing the Standards

The next phase in the development of the standard, after the conceptual standards assessment, was the development of the *interoperability standard*. This is where the actual standard development work is drafted to refine the standards selected in the conceptual standards assessment, adjusting the chosen base standards to address Ontario-specific requirements, where the business requirements of the solution dictate adjustment is needed. The format of the standard closely follows the format used by Canada Health Infoway and the international standards development organizations (SDOs). The specifications drafted included guiding documentation to support the implementation and sustained use of DI CS. The interoperability standards assessment is completed with the drafting of the specifications, and this includes providing details about the data model and interactions used in the standard, with a focus on the logical application layer. This and other published EHR interoperability standards are available through eHealth Ontario (eHealth Ontario 2008–2016).

Standards in DI CS

The Cross-Enterprise Document Sharing (XDS.b) profile from IHE has become the industry standard mechanism for sharing documents between institutions, and the Cross-Enterprise Document Sharing for Imaging (XDS-I.b) supplement to this profile extends XDS to share images, diagnostic reports, and related information across a group of care sites. In Canada, the most widely implemented messaging standard in healthcare organizations is a standard called HL7 V2 (HL7 FAQ n.d.). HL7 V2 was first developed in 1989 and is a fairly simple and efficient standard, designed mostly to support workflows inside a hospital and not between organizations. In the 1990s, HL7 developed a new standard, HL7 V3, based on object-oriented modeling principals and the simple object access protocol messaging exchange, which followed a much more complex data model and allowed for much more detailed collection of coded data. This included the CDA, a standard based on HL7 V3 for specifying how clinical documents should be constructed. While some organizations are using HL7 V3, many have not had a strong incentive to move from HL7 V2 based on its prevalent use in the United States and preexisting systems across healthcare settings in Canada since the early 1990s. There is also little appetite to move to a new standard while hospital budgets are constrained. Most healthcare settings in Ontario are still using HL7 V2 for DI and other clinical reports, and this limits the ability to have discrete data available that can be interpreted by other systems and used for analytical purposes in future. Having this more detailed discrete data could provide more valuable insights into the performance metrics and outcomes for DI in Ontario. Health service providers are focused on delivering healthcare, and the time needed to manage the migration to a new standard can add additional stress to a healthcare system with limited resources and an aging population. This and a number of healthcare organizations with large volumes of DI reports and manifests add to the complexity and challenges of moving to a new standard. The DI CS standard use of a document-based infrastructure using XDS-I provides a way to take these basic messages and include them in the document-based architecture, paving the way to using basic CDA documents and to using more sophisticated discrete data in the future.

Cross-Enterprise Document Sharing

XDS is a specification for allowing a group of organizations that have agreed to exchange information (called an Affinity Domain) to submit documents for sharing through a centralized infrastructure. It defines a set of systems capabilities or *actors* and related transactions to allow systems to submit documents to the sharing infrastructure and to query them back, using a defined set of metadata items describing the type of document, the source of the document, and the patient the document relates to. Any computer system that has all of the capabilities of the actor, and can perform all of the transactions associated with it, is said to *implement* that actor.

Central to this sharing infrastructure is an actor called an XDS Registry. This registry holds all of the metadata about the documents available to be queried, a list of known patients, as well as links to the actual location of the documents. An Affinity Domain can only have one XDS Registry and it serves as the central coordinating point for the sharing of documents.

In order for the XDS Registry to have a list of known patients, it has to have a place to get information about the patients, which is an actor known as the Patient Identity Source. A Patient Identity Source has one transaction, the Patient Identity Feed, also known as ITI-8 (all IHE transactions have numbers as well as names), which feeds information about the patients in the Affinity Domain to the XDS Registry.

Systems that implement the Document Source actor are able to submit documents to the central infrastructure, along with the appropriate metadata. We also need an accessible place to store the documents, known as an XDS Repository. Unlike the XDS Registry, there can be any number of these and, depending on the architecture chosen and the rules for sharing set up by the Affinity Domain, they are sometimes combined with the Document Source in a single system. If combined, they use a single transaction called a Register Document Set (ITI-42), which sends the metadata to the registry. If separate, the Document Source sends a Provide and Register Document Set (ITI-41) transaction to the repository, which triggers the registration process.

The final piece of the XDS puzzle is the Document Consumer, which is an actor or system that can query the XDS Registry for a list of documents, using a Registry Stored Query (ITI-18) transaction, and then retrieve those documents from a repository. The Registry Stored Query transaction supports a number of different kinds of queries, all based on the document metadata. Examples include querying by patient ID, for a specific time range, by author, and by the type of document. Finally, a Retrieve Document Set (ITI-43) transaction allows the consuming system to fetch the documents and display them to the end user. The infrastructure is depicted in Figure 6.8.

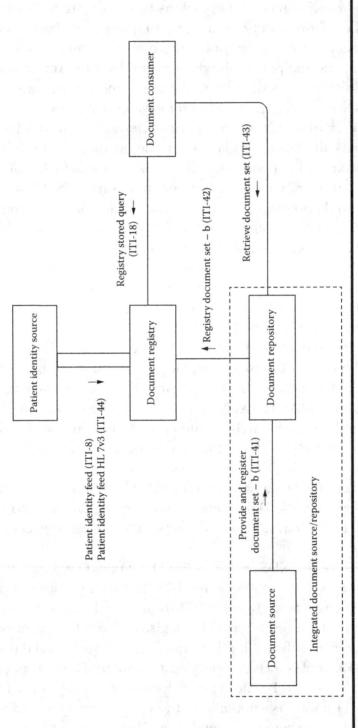

Figure 6.8 XDS infrastructure diagram. (From IHE International Inc. n.d. IHE IT Infrastructure Technical Framework. IHE. http://www.ihe.net/uploadedFiles/Documents/ITI/IHE_ITI_TF_Vol1.pdf.)

XDS Affinity Domain

Underlying this infrastructure is the Affinity Domain. When organizations are making agreements to share information, there are a number of items that have to be considered, from policy and procedure questions such as access rights for different types of users and what types of data are considered sensitive, to technical considerations such as how backups are done and what type of encryption to use.

When setting up an XDS Affinity Domain, there are two key technical considerations. The first is what patient identifier is going to be used as the single authoritative unique ID for the patient. In the case of eHealth Ontario, this was already determined by the blueprint. The unique ID assigned to the patient in the Client Registry is, by definition, the unique ID for all eHealth Ontario projects, and the Client Registry would be our Patient Identity Source actor.

The second consideration is more complex, and that is the determination of what values would be allowed for the XDS Registry metadata fields. Some of these metadata fields are free text, like the document title, and can be determined by each individual organization in the Affinity Domain without affecting the others, but there are some fields that must be restricted to certain values that all organizations in the Affinity Domain agree on if the system is going to work. The most important of these are the *values*, or *codes*, that define the type of document.

- classCode: A high-level classification for the kind of document it is—for example report, image, or workflow
- eventCodeList: A list of codes describing the main clinical events being documented
- healthcareFacilityTypeCode: The kind of facility where the clinical encounter occurred—for example, hospital, outpatient clinic, or primary care office
- practiceSettingCode: The specialty of the setting where the procedures being documented occurred—for example, radiology, laboratory, or cardiology
- typeCode: A code for the specific type of document being recorded, more fine-grained than the classCode—for example, *echocardiogram report* rather than simply *report*

In order for document sharing to work, for Document Sources to be able to submit documents, and for Document Consumers to be able to query for them and get the correct results, everyone has to be using the same values for these fields. This is usually done by defining value sets for each metadata element, selecting the codes in each value set from a particular terminology. However, most existing systems already have their own value sets and use their own terminologies. In order to integrate these systems into DI CS, a set of mappings had to be produced, to provide translations from the value sets used in the local environments to those used inside the DI CS system. The process by which the value sets were chosen and the mappings completed is explained in more detail in the section "Terminology Standards."

Extensions for Imaging

Since XDS was created for sharing documents, and the DI CS project was created to share imaging studies and reports, a few alterations have to be made to the base XDS profile, both to the actors and transactions and to the types of metadata associated with the documents. These alterations are contained in the XDS-I profile from IHE's radiology domain.

The first addition that has to be made is to the actors and transactions for XDS. In addition to those already discussed, XDS-I adds an Imaging Document Source and an Imaging Document Consumer. The profile makes some changes to the Provide and Register Document Set transaction, introducing the very similar Provide and Register Imaging Document Set transaction in its place, which introduces changes to the metadata to accommodate images and imaging documents. The changes made on the Document Consumer side are more extensive. Aside from the corresponding Retrieve Imaging Document Set that accommodates the same metadata changes as the Provide and Register transaction, the Imaging Document Consumer adds six new transactions that use Digital Imaging and Communications in Medicine (DICOM) protocols to fetch DICOM image files, Key Image Note files, and other kinds of imaging-specific document types (Figure 6.9).

XDS-I also made changes to the definition and content of some of the metadata fields, to be able to include some key pieces of data that are not used routinely outside of the DI field. In some cases, this involved overriding the base meaning of the field, and in others, it involved adding new fields not included in XDS.

Two pieces of data that are extremely important in DI but not commonly used in other areas of practice, are the *imaging modality* (whether the images

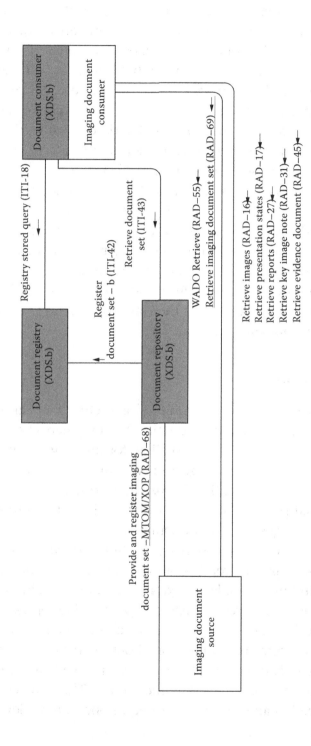

Figure 6.9 **XDS Extensions for Imaging. (From Integrating the Healthcare Enterprise (IHE). 2008–2016. Cross-Enterprise Document Sharing for Imaging. http://wiki.ihe.net/index.php/Cross-enterprise_Document_Sharing_for_Imaging.**

were taken by x-ray, CT scan, MRI, etc.) and the *region of anatomy* in the images. The radiology domain, when writing XDS-I, decided to repurpose the eventList field to contain the codes for modality and anatomy. The procedure code, which normally would be contained in eventList, is moved to the typeCode. In implementations that handle both imaging and nonimaging documents, this difference in the placement of procedure codes can cause significant confusion if not closely managed; however, in the case of DI CS, only imaging artifacts are considered and eHealth Ontario can ignore the conflict.

The other metadata change of note is the addition of a field called *referenceIdList*, which is used to store an identifier called the Accession Number. The Accession Number is very important in DI. It is assigned when an order for an imaging study is issued and is carried through to the entire radiology workflow, from scheduling to image acquisition, storage, image review, and finally report. It allows clinicians to unequivocally relate the images to the report. This field was not included in XDS when the radiology domain first wrote XDS-I and was added as a special metadata slot. While XDS did eventually incorporate the referenceIdList in their metadata, many vendors have not yet updated their implementations.

Clinical Document Architecture

At this point, we have a document-sharing infrastructure that can uniquely identify the patient, can appropriately identify the documents with consistent metadata, and has been extended to allow for imaging documents and images, as well as general reports. However, we still have an abundance of source systems that are using HL7 V2, instead of documents, to transmit their reports. The final piece of the DI CS technical infrastructure is a way to translate those V2 messages into CDA documents.

The CDA is an HL7 standard for exchanging clinical documents, such as discharge summaries, diagnostic reports or operative notes, using XML. CDA documents all contain human-readable text and can also contain images and multimedia content, as well as coded, machine-processable representations of information. All CDA documents consist of a document header and a document body. The header contains information about the patient's demographics, the event the document is recording, the clinicians involved, and other metadata that describe the contents of the document body. The body contains the actual clinical information and can be formatted in one of three levels.

1. Level 1 CDA documents have a document body that is unstructured. That is to say, it is something other than XML formatted content. This could be a scan of a PDF, an image, or just plain text.
2. Level 2 CDA documents have a body that is XML based, and consists of a number of *sections*, each of which contains narrative text.
3. Level 3 CDA documents are also in XML, and contain sections, along with entries, that contain coded, machine-processable information that describes the contents for the narrative text (Figure 6.10).

As the level of the document body increases, so does the level of interoperability and semantics in the data. At Level 1, the body is completely unstructured and, while it is readable and understandable by a human, the amount of information that can be interpreted by the computer systems and applications that are exchanging the data is limited. The introduction of sections at Level 2 allows the systems to determine the type of information contained in each portion of the documents (i.e., drugs the patient is taking in the "Medications" section, allergies and sensitivities in the "Allergies" section), and finally, the introduction of fully coded entries at Level 3 allows for the detailed processing of the clinical information in the document by the systems involved.

For full semantic interoperability (i.e., the ability for the systems involved in data exchange to completely parse and interpret the data), Level 3 CDA documents are required. However, many systems still in use today are not capable of transmitting these fully coded documents, and many systems are still using HL7 V2 messages, which, as was mentioned previously, do not lend themselves well to fully coded data. Having the three different levels of CDA documents allows a phased approach to interoperability, with each system contributing data at the highest level of which it is capable.

In the case of DI CS, the submitting systems were all using an HL7 V2 Observation Result (ORU) message to submit radiology reports. The lack of coded and structured data in these messages meant that when we translated these messages into CDA, we were restricted to a Level 1 format, with no structured, coded data. However, the choice to use CDA allows for a progression to more complex data formats as the contributing systems gain those capabilities, without the need for significant rework of the main infrastructure.

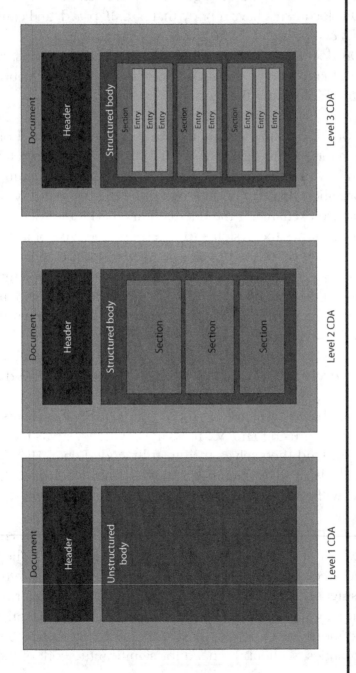

Figure 6.10   The three levels of CDA.

Terminology Standards

As we described previously, terminologies and vocabularies, and the ability to map between them, are key components of being able to share and interpret clinical information. Establishing the terminology standards for the DI CS initiative began with involvement from Canada Health Infoway, eHealth Ontario, clinical stakeholders from the four regional DI-rs, and Mohawk Shared Services, the regional partner organization charged with the terminology standards definition and development (Figure 6.7). The scope of the DI CS project terminology standards is highlighted in Table 6.2. The working group formed by these organizations reported to a steering committee with representation from Canada Health Infoway, Mohawk Shared Services, and eHealth Ontario. Some examples of the type of guidance provided are decisions about what the XDS (IHE 2008–2016) metadata would include, what the terminology set would include, how the terminology set and maps would be validated, what the local-to-provincial terminology maps would include, and what the process would be for adding to the terminology set.

Education of the working group membership regarding standards, especially terminology standards and related supporting browsers and mapping tools, became important to the overall success of the project. A common

Table 6.2 Terminology Standards Scope

In Scope	Out of Scope
• Creation of an Ontario DI terminology set that is to be mapped to SNOMED CT • Definition of terminology-mapping rules and the creation of documentation to support the mapping of local terms • Provision of assistance to hospitals across Ontario to map their local terms to the Ontario DI terminology • Implementation of a governance model and policies for the maintenance and support of the terminology set, maps, and related documentation • Education of stakeholders in the creation, communications, and implementation of the terminology	• Mapping of the DI codes to the Canadian Institute for Health Information (CIHI) Management Information System (MIS) codes • Mapping of the DI codes to the Ontario Health Insurance Plan Billing codes • Mapping of the DI codes to the CIHI Canadian Classification of Health Interventions (CCI) codes • Development of the pan-Canadian DI terminology set (However, the work done by this project can become a foundation for the Canadian DI terminology.) • Translation of Ontario DI terminology into French

understanding of the terminology use options, and the decisions that needed to be made about the format, structure, and use of the terminology standards in the solution, all assisted the working group with the completion of the terminology standards scope activities, as shown in Table 6.2. Because the regional DI-rs were already in use in some regions, the clinical representatives were able to share the approach implemented or being implemented for the regional DI-rs, including the sharing of the regional terminology set terms, local-to-regional maps, mapping lessons learned, and insights regarding terminology practices and tools, such as Apelon Termworks (n.d.).

The comprehensive terminology assessment completed in the early stages of the project was the comparison of terminology standards that could be used to represent the DI procedures in a provincial terminology list. This terminology standards assessment included a comparison of SNOMED CT, a comprehensive, multilingual clinical healthcare terminology that enables consistent, processable representation of clinical content in EHRs with a procedures hierarchy covering DI procedures (SNOMED International 2016) and RadLex®, a comprehensive unified language of radiology terms for the standardized indexing and retrieval of radiology information resources (RSNA 2016). eHealth Ontario determined that SNOMED CT best met the business requirements and specific terminology needs for the DI CS project and aligned with Ontario's eHealth Blueprint (eHealth Ontario 2014). This decision was based on the status of RadLex Version 3.4 at the time this work was commencing (2011; Version 3.13 was released in November 2015) (RSNA 2008–2015) and the timelines for the eHealth Ontario DI CS initiative. Consultation with Canada Health Infoway and Mohawk Shared Services, with contacts from the Radiological Society of North America (RSNA) (RSNA 2016) involved in the development of RadLex and the United Kingdom's Terminology Centre involved in the UK implementation of DI procedure terminology standards (NHS 2016), all helped inform the final recommended approach. The preparation for the standards development work included research into other DI projects with a similar approach to using a DI procedure code system or standard DI procedure names. Projects in Canada and other countries were assessed through interviews with contacts to understand the scope and purpose of the use of terminology in the project. This opportunity to discuss the work implemented elsewhere provided valuable insights into experiences and knowledge that helped inform the decision-making and direction of the DI CS project.

One of the key terminology decisions that had to be made was in the use of precoordination or postcoordination of code sets. Postcoordination and precoordination are different ways of handling code sets where the full description of a concept requires multiple dimensions. In DI CS, the dimensions in question were codes to represent the procedure done, the laterality (side of the body) of the procedure, the type of imaging modality used, and the anatomical site. In postcoordination, the codes would be used separately and then linked together to fully describe the procedure. To use precoordination, the dimensions would be combined in advance and used as a single concept. As an example, suppose you wanted to encode "CT scan, right knee." To express this using postcoordination, "CT scan" (modality), "right side" (laterality), and "knee" (anatomy) would all be recorded separately. To get a full description of the procedure performed, the codes would need to be combined when the scan is read. Precoordination would involve combining the terms and assigning a single code to the concept "CT scan, right knee." To use precoordination, all possible combinations of all these dimensions would need to be determined in advance and an individual code assigned to each combination, which would add codes not included in the international version of SNOMED CT (SNOMED International 2016).

SNOMED CT developed over time through requests for additions to the SDO, and there were some variations used in naming DI procedures in SNOMED CT that the DI CS project team felt could compromise adoption in vendor systems, the use for navigation in the viewer, and with foreign exam management in the future. With input from clinicians and terminology and technical experts, a precoordination approach was decided on, and a user interface code and term for each DI procedure was created using a consistent naming format that included the DI procedure with the modality, body part, laterality, and use of contrast. SNOMED CT was mapped to the user interface code and term to allow eHealth Ontario to use SNOMED CT in the provincial solution for DI CS, resulting in the creation of a provincial terminology set for DI procedures. About 2500 concepts were submitted to Canada Health Infoway as requests for change requiring assessment for inclusion in the international core release of SNOMED CT, resulting in many new concepts available for use in Canada and internationally. Canada Health Infoway works with SNOMED International (formerly International Health Terminology Standards Development Organization [IHTSDO]). to minimize the number of concepts remaining in the Canadian extension of SNOMED CT. eHealth Ontario has completed the update of the additions with the corresponding SNOMED CT codes and descriptions received to date, and

Table 6.3 eHealth Ontario DI Terminology Components

eHealth Ontario DI Terminology Components	eHealth Ontario DI Terminology Description
Ontario DI terminology set	Terminology set of DI procedures for representing DI results in Ontario's DI CS
Ontario user interface term identifier	Ontario code used to identify the Ontario equivalent of the DI procedure for each DI result
Ontario user interface term description	Ontario description used to identify the Ontario equivalent of the DI procedure for each DI result, including modality, body part, laterality, and contrast
SNOMED CT concept identifier	SNOMED CT code used to identify the DI procedure for each DI result
SNOMED CT fully specified name	SNOMED CT description used to identify the DI procedure for each DI result
SNOMED CT concept identifier—Canadian extension	SNOMED CT code used to identify the DI procedure for each DI result
SNOMED CT fully specified name—Canadian extension	SNOMED CT description used to identify the DI procedure for each DI result

expects to continue to receive additions with continuing implementations. In future, eHealth Ontario expects to submit the occasional request for additions as DI procedures are added based on technological changes and innovations. Table 6.3 illustrates the Ontario DI terminology set components.

Implementation

In order to better manage such a large-scale project, the DI program developed an iterative implementation approach where each release incrementally increased in functionality until the future state vision was achieved. The rationale for a phased implementation included the following:

■ Faster implementation than a single release of the fully developed future state
■ Faster realization of clinical benefits

■ Increased ability for feedback from healthcare providers' actual use in the clinical environment back into the design, construction, and functionality of subsequent releases

■ Increased ability to leverage shared services as they become available— for example, terminology services or consent management

More specifically, the releases were divided in the following manner:

■ Release 1 enables province-wide access to diagnostic reports through web portals, beginning with the eHealth Ontario portal.

■ Release 2 enables the sharing and access of DI images stored in the four DI-rs across Ontario using a *provincial viewer* and sets the foundation for future releases.

■ Future releases would be based on adoption and demand and would include EMR-based access and PACS-based access, as well as other points of service as required, to fulfill the intent of providing clinicians with access channels best suited to their workflow.

During the planning stages of the DI CS initiative, there were two main options being considered.

1. One XDS Registry with four XDS Repositories (one per DI-r)
2. One XDS Registry with one XDS Repository

The XDS Registry was already being procured by eHealth Ontario as part of the provincial HIAL initiative, so that element was resolved. However, the repository component still required an approach. Early in the project, the decision was made to use the existing regional DI-rs instead of creating a single, consolidated repository at eHealth Ontario and duplicating the content from the four DI-rs. This approach was determined to be the most effective for access across the province to the volume of reports and images needed to support the population in Ontario (over 13 million residents) and also takes advantage of the XDS-I standard, which is supported by all of the regional repositories. As the business requirements for the DI CS solution were refined, the procurement of the DI CS solution focused on specifying the hardware, software, and interoperability standards.

At that time, that approach made sense because

■ The status quo of the DI-rs as both document and image archives would be maintained.
■ The DI-rs were being upgraded anyway and XDS functionality would be available (although the purchase of licenses would be required).
■ eHealth Ontario would implement the central XDS Registry as part of the HIAL.

However, throughout 2012, the DI-r vendors were slow to complete upgrades, preventing the implementation of XDS. Ultimately, eHealth Ontario procured one XDS Registry as part of its HIAL implementation and one XDS Repository thereby eliminating the need for multiple assets across the province. This centralized model placed clear accountability on eHealth Ontario to implement the registry and repository while simultaneously ensuring cost containment and the reduction of complexity. One of the consequences of vendors being slow to implement upgrades is the lack of support for certain features of more advanced XDS implementation. While the systems procured by eHealth Ontario had support for all of the functionality of XDS, even those systems lacked support for more recent additions, such as support for the metadata updates necessary to support patient link change events.

Patient link changes occur when it is determined that two separate patient records in the system actually belong to the same person. The Client Registry uses two types of identifiers for a patient: a universal ID that uniquely identifies a single patient and a set of local medical record numbers (MRNs). A patient can have multiple MRNs, depending on how many healthcare facilities they have been to, but should have only one single universal ID. The patient's many MRNs are "linked" to the universal ID. A link change occurs when we have to alter the universal ID that a given MRN is attached to.

When documents are sent to an XDS Repository and the metadata is sent to the registry, two of the fields that are required are the universal ID for the patient, and the local MRN. When a link change occurs in the Client Registry, it's necessary for that change to also be made in the XDS Registry, or the possibility exists that queries will bring back information for the wrong patient. The preferred way to do that is using an IHE profile for XDS Affinity Domain Patient Identifier Change Management (XAD-PID), which specifies a way for changes in patient links at the Client Registry level to be propagated to other systems in the Affinity Domain, including the XDS Registry. However, as this is a relatively new profile, many of the systems in the eHealth Ontario ecosystem don't have this capability.

To provide the necessary updates, the DI program decided to use the capabilities of the HIAL to mimic the XAD-PID functionality. Every time the HIAL was notified of a patient link change event in the Client Registry, it constructed and sent a Update Document Set (ITI-57) message to the registry, which included the new universal ID and the MRN for which the change was being made, which allowed the XDS Registry to make the necessary corrections.

One other issue around patient link changes occurred when it was noticed that some of the end-user systems were keeping a record of the patient's universal ID, rather than querying for it each time they wanted to obtain records, and as they weren't getting updates when the patient links changed, they were using outdated information to make their queries. Once again, the HIAL functionality provided the solution to the problem, allowing us to intercept the request, query the Client Registry for the correct identifier, and replace the information in the request with the updated information before sending it on to the registry.

The implementation of the privacy and security strategy is now complete. Integration with the eHealth Ontario central authentication and authorization solution, ONE ID, is complete, ensuring consistent and robust access control to the PHI contained in the DI CS solution. Translation of the Audit Trail and Node Authentication (ATNA) audit messages produced by the XDS solution to the format required by the eHealth Ontario central audit repository is also complete, and an end-to-end audit trace of system access is available. One other important addition to DI CS that is also now complete is the application of a provincial patient consent solution. Early in the implementation, DI CS had a basic consent solution applied to it based on the IHE Basic Patient Privacy and Consent profile. The upgrade of the consent solution was integral to the overall privacy and security strategy of eHealth Ontario and has allowed the enforcement of detailed consent policies and consent override at a provincial level. eHealth Ontario developed a comprehensive consent model and specification in 2012, and the implementation of the related solution was completed in 2016, at which time, DI CS was switched over to the provincial solution (Figure 6.11).

Future State

The current state of the DI CS initiative is delivering radiology reports and images to providers across the province of Ontario, but there are a few things to be done to complete the project.

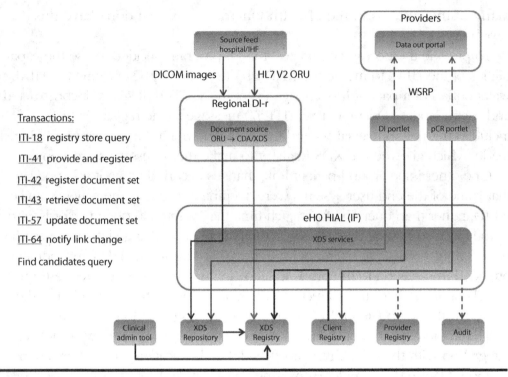

Transactions:

ITI-18 registry store query

ITI-41 provide and register

ITI-42 register document set

ITI-43 retrieve document set

ITI-57 update document set

ITI-64 notify link change

Find candidates query

Figure 6.11   XDS-I data flow with metadata update. (From © eHealth Ontario 2015, reprinted with permission, eHealth Ontario 2017.)

The largest of these was to complete the integration of the project with the second iteration of the Ontario HIAL to enable the full range of HIAL features. With the new HIAL in place, the upgrade to the complete privacy and security framework and the provincial consent solution were implemented in 2016. The implementation of the runtime full set of terminology mappings is the other work planned for the new HIAL; the terminology component of the project is now in progress in 2017.

The terminology maps have been verified, and some additional terminology maps will be added in the coming year with the addition of more IHFs and changes to some of the existing hospital systems. The terminology mapping work has been maintained over the course of the project and is very close to testing with the DI CS solution; it is then planned to be used in HIAL 2.0 with DI CS and the eHealth Ontario DI Viewer. The terminology will be applied at runtime in the viewer to support the more precise selection of reports and image manifests. As more diagnostic studies from more contributing organizations are added to DI CS, the value of a common terminology to describe the DI procedure consistently across the repository will be important for the effective presentation of the correct DI studies for the patient. Future work with *foreign exam management*, or the import of DI exams from other DI systems for comparative use in a DI system, is also expected to demonstrate clinical benefit through the consistent use of common terminology for the DI procedure, modality, and body part.

Conclusion

The effective implementation of complex integration projects requires input from a variety of stakeholders with a variety of skillsets. While the technical expertise in standards and terminologies is valuable, it is vital to get input early on in the project from the clinical professionals that will actually be using and relying on the system, to ensure that the solution provided works within the clinical domain. This collaboration should be continued throughout the life of the project and during the ongoing maintenance of the standards, maps, and terminology sets, to ensure that clinicians' work is supported as the standards and solutions evolve.

Standards should be selected using criteria to ensure the best fit for business needs, both current and future. The purpose of the standards, the criteria to define what is "fit for use" by systems, and the format, structure, and standards management practices to be used must be defined early on, and flexibility must be addressed for future changes.

Differences in the data standards in use in the systems contributing to the integrations will influence your solution design and the ability to share information among systems. Changes or upgrades to the contributing systems can result in the need for substantial modifications to support the new systems. Build maintenance and change management procedures into your standards framework early on and address any concerns with vendors early and often.

Finally, when undertaking a complex integration project, it is important to engage directly with the SDOs that are responsible for the standards that will be central to your project. They are an invaluable source of early guidance, lessons learned, and knowledge of purpose, use, and toolsets to support their standards. At the end of the implementation, you can contribute back to the SDO for future releases of the standards, which may benefit from content from other implementers (Table 6.4).

Table 6.4   Learning Opportunities Identified (eHealth Ontario 2014)

Category	Description	Opportunity
Clinical and Technical Expertise	• *Clinical advice* from DI domain subject matter experts, radiologists, primary care physicians, and other clinical professionals who actually rely on the DI reports and images. • *Mapping guidance* by terminology experts who understand the terminology rules and how the terminology standard is applied in the solution. • *Standards guidance* by technical experts with input from terminology experts, DI domain subject matter experts, and technical implementers who understand the standard, the solution, and the use of the data collected in the solution.	• Understand the *options and limitations* from the specific domain, clinical, technical, and terminology perspectives. • Continue *collaboration* for accurate quality in the *ongoing maintenance* of standards, maps, and the terminology set, including local dictionary changes to DI procedures, modalities, and anatomy. • *Enhance and evolve the solution and use of standards* with early and continued engagement to address requirements and ensure the solution is well supported by the standards selected and as they evolve in future.
Standards Selection	• *Standards selection* using criteria to inform the best selection for the business requirements, solution, and alignment across the EHR (eHealth Ontario 2013).	• Select the *best standards* to meet the needs, best fit, available options, and any potential future plans for the intended purpose or use of the data collected in the solution (e.g., direct care, population health, and other data analytics) with consideration of policy and regulation.

(Continued)

Table 6.4 (Continued)   Learning Opportunities Identified (eHealth Ontario 2014)

Category	Description	Opportunity
Standards Management	• *Define standards purpose, use by systems, format, structure and standards management practices early,* with consideration of local and health information exchange solutions and *flexibility for future change.* • Leverage the *right standards tools;* determine what you need to manage, map, maintain, and comply with the standards and the best possible tools and practices available.	• Obtain *early guidance with questions and decisions* from *standards organizations* for added expertise and *document all decisions* regarding structure, format, purpose, use, and tools, including any attributes required to support specific needs, rationale, definitions, terminology set, maps, guiding principles, and standards maintenance practices. • *Address compliance with standards* in the solution with regular touch points during interface development, implementation of the solution, validation of data quality, and testing for standards compliance from contributing sources. • *Contribute to the future standards releases* for international standards that may benefit from content needed by others.
Solution Design and Interoperability	• *Different data standards in RIS and PACS can influence your solution* design and ability to share information from local to health information exchange systems. • *Changes* to RIS or PACS dictionaries, vendors, solutions, or standards will impact the application of standards and may result in a need to adapt the solution to support the changes.	• *Address any concerns early* with vendors, systems users, and standards organizations that may impact how you can design, use, and evolve systems. • *Understand your options* for standards in the solution and with complementary systems, such as terminology knowledge bases used at runtime to enhance the navigation of search results by DI procedure, modality, and anatomy. • Build in *maintenance processes to ensure your solution is able to evolve with changes,* including combining RIS or PACS dictionaries across multiple organizations and updates to international standards, and local terminology changes.

References

Apelon Termworks. n.d. Terminology Tooling Products. http://www.apelon.com/solutions/terminology-tooling/termworks.

Better Outcomes Registry and Network (BORN). 2016. BORN Ontario. https://www.bornontario.ca/ (accessed Nov. 2, 2016).

Canada Health Infoway. n.d. EHRS Blueprint v2 Fact Sheet. https://www.infoway-inforoute.ca/en/component/edocman/194-an-ehrs-blueprint-v2-fact-sheet/view-document?Itemid=101 (accessed Nov. 2, 2016).

Canada Health Infoway. 2016. Projects List. https://www.infoway-inforoute.ca/en/what-we-do/progress-in-canada/investment-programs (accessed Nov. 2, 2016).

Canadian Institute for Health Information. 2014. National Health Expenditure Trends 1975 to 2014. October. https://www.cihi.ca/en/nhex_2014_report_en.pdf.

Canadian Press. 2015. *CBC News Politics.* Nov 9. http://www.cbc.ca/news/politics/5-things-to-know-about-the-liberal-pledge-to-establish-a-new-health-accord-1.3311464 (accessed Nov. 9, 2015).

eHealth Ontario. 2008–2016. EHR Connectivity Strategy. http://www.ehealthontario.on.ca/en/ehr-connectivity-strategy (accessed Nov. 2, 2016).

eHealth Ontario. 2008–2016. Ontario EHR Interoperability Standards. http://www.ehealthontario.on.ca/en/architecture/standards (accessed Nov. 2, 2016).

eHealth Ontario. 2013. Standards Selection Guide. *eHealth Ontario.* http://www.ehealthontario.on.ca/images/uploads/pages/documents/eHealth_Standards_Selection_Framework_en.pdf (accessed Nov. 2, 2016).

eHealth Ontario. 2014. Ontario's eHealth Blueprint In-Depth. *eHealth Ontario.* http://www.ehealthblueprint.com/assets/documentation/Blueprint_Book.pdf.

eHealth Ontario. 2014. Terminology Lessons—Jurisdictional View. *eHealth Ontario.* http://www.e-healthconference.com/pastpresentations/2015/201462029909/eHealthOntario_eHealth2014_2014_06_03_Final.pdf (accessed Oct. 26, 2016).

eHealth Ontario. 2015. Benefits Realization Update, 2015. eHealth Ontario. http://www.ehealthontario.on.ca/images/uploads/annual_reports/Benefits_Realization_Update-en.pdf.

Government of Canada. 2017. Canada reaches health funding agreement with Ontario. Health Canada. March 10. https://www.canada.ca/en/health-canada/news/2017/03/canada_reaches_healthfundingagreementwithontario.html.

Health Level Seven (HL7). 2005. Product Brief: Clinical Document Architecture Release 2. May. http://www.hl7.org/implement/standards/product_brief.cfm?product_id=7 (accessed Nov. 2, 2016).

HL7 FAQ. n.d. http://www.hl7.org/about/FAQs/index.cfm?ref=nav.

IHE International Inc. n.d. IHE IT Infrastructure Technical Framework. IHE. http://www.ihe.net/uploadedFiles/Documents/ITI/IHE_ITI_TF_Vol1.pdf.

Integrating the Healthcare Enterprise (IHE). 2008–2016. Cross-Enterprise Document Sharing for Imaging. http://wiki.ihe.net/index.php/Cross-enterprise_Document_Sharing_for_Imaging. (accessed Nov. 2, 2016).

Mohwak Shared Services Inc. 2016. Mohawk Shared Service Inc.—Diagnostic Imaging Repostitory. https://www.mohawkssi.com/en/services/diagnosticimag-ingrepository.asp (accessed Nov. 2, 2016).

NHS. 2016. National Interim Clinical Imaging Procedure (NICIP) Code Set. Oct 26. http://www.datadictionary.nhs.uk/web_site_content/supporting_informa-tion/clinical_coding/national_interim_clinical_imaging_procedure_code_set. asp?shownav=1 (accessed Nov. 2, 2016).

Ontario MD. 2015. Ontario MD Annual Report. *Ontario MD.* https://www. ontariomd.ca/portal/server.pt/community/our_organization/731/ annual_reports/24343.

Ontario Ministry of Health and Long-Term Care (MOHLTC). n.d. Health Services in Your Community. http://www.health.gov.on.ca/en/common/system/services/.

RSNA. 2008–2015. RadLex Release Notes. *Google Docs.* https://docs.google. com/document/d/10zRIBkXyj1eLt3LS_A7w3gSGRedXXoYvucH6H4trCZY/ edit?hl=en&pref=2&pli=1 (accessed Nov. 2, 2016).

RSNA. 2016. Radiological Society of North America—RadLex: What Is RadLex? http://www.rsna.org/RadLex.aspx (accessed Nov. 2, 2016).

RSNA. 2016. Radiological Society of North America—About RSNA. http://www.rsna. org/AboutRSNA.aspx (accessed Nov. 2, 2016).

SNOMED International. 2016. International Health Terminology Standards Development Organization—What Is It? http://www.ihtsdo.org/snomed-ct/ what-is-snomed-ct (accessed Nov. 2, 2016).

Chapter 7

E-Vital Standards Initiative

Michelle Williamson and Hetty Khan

Contents

Introduction

The National Vital Statistics System (NVSS) is a premier example of intergovernmental data sharing in public health.* It supports the collection of vital records data, including births, fetal deaths, and deaths, and the dissemination of official vital statistics. Vital statistics data impact national health and healthcare-related policy decisions and influence programmatic and policy

---

* Centers for Disease Control and Prevention. (2015). National Vital Statistics System: About the National Vital Statistics System. Retrieved from: http://www.cdc.gov/nchs/nvss/about_nvss.htm.

decisions for state agencies.* The vital statistics community has been collaborating to support a National Center for Health Statistics (NCHS) initiative to enhance data collection processes by exploring the use of electronic health record (EHR) systems to capture medical and health information for vital statistics purposes, with the aim of improving the timeliness, accuracy, and quality of the data. The increase in EHR adoption in the United States provides an opportunity for the integration of information and improved data sharing. Such integration and data sharing can potentially improve public health's ability to monitor the health of the nation and the healthcare system and to link data in multiple ways for a healthier population. Standards are the essential building blocks for EHRs and enable data sharing and comparability.

The NCHS e-Vital Standards Initiative is focused on developing an electronic, standards-based approach for vital records data collection using health information technology (HIT) standards. Accomplishing this goal requires stakeholder engagement with key vital records stakeholders, standards development organizations (SDOs), and EHR and vital record system vendors. A major component also involves the development of HIT standards with a specific focus on including vital records requirements. This chapter will provide an overview of the NVSS. Additionally, it will elaborate on the collaborations that have occurred among key stakeholders and the chronological standards development activities that have contributed to the e-Vital Standards Initiative.

Overview of the National Vital Statistics System

In the United States, the NVSS is the mechanism by which the nation collects official records of vital events such as live births, fetal deaths, deaths, marriages, and divorces.† The NVSS is a cooperative system between individual states and federal agencies supported by the Vital Statistics Cooperative Program (VSCP) and administered by the Centers for Disease Control and Preventions' NCHS. Through the VSCP, NCHS contracts with

---

* Centers for Disease Control and Prevention. (2012). CDC Healthcare Information Management Systems Society 2012 white paper: CDC connecting to healthcare through interoperability. Retrieved from: http://www.cdc.gov/nchs/data/dvs/evital/14-CDC-HIMSS-2012-Interoperability-White-Paper.pdf.

† O'Carroll, P., Yasnoff, W., Ward, E., Ripp, L., and Martin, E. (2003). *Public Health Informatics and Information Systems*. New York: Springer.

individual states and jurisdictions to establish the mechanism by which data are collected from state vital registration systems and national vital statistics disseminated.*

Dating back to the twentieth century, the legal authority for the registration of live births, fetal deaths, and deaths has resided with the states, official jurisdictions (New York City and Washington, DC), and territories (Puerto Rico, the US Virgin Islands, Guam, American Samoa, and the Commonwealth of the Northern Mariana Islands) in which the event occurred.† The states are responsible for the registration of all vital events based on state laws and for issuing certificates and records to individuals. Statistical information (demographic, medical, and geographic) is derived from over 4 million birth certificates and about 2.4 million death certificates and fetal death reports.‡

In the United States, reporting requirements for birth, fetal death, and death vary from state to state. In hospitals and birthing centers, the attendant at birth (e.g., physician or midwife) reports the birth event to the state or jurisdictional vital records office by completing a birth certificate. The jurisdiction has the authority to register the birth after it has been reported. Fetal deaths are reported by the completion of a fetal death report. Fetal deaths are spontaneous intrauterine deaths at any time during the pregnancy, but are generally presented in vital statistics information for fetal deaths of 20 weeks' gestation or more.§ For deaths, responsibility for reporting typically resides with the funeral director, who will obtain the decedent's information from the family and initiate the death certificate. Completion of the death certificate, however, is a responsibility shared with the medical certifier who completes the *cause of death* section. The medical certifier may be a physician or medical examiner/coroner, depending on the circumstances of the death.¶

Although the registration of vital record events is a legal requirement of the state and protects the rights of individual citizens, the importance of collecting such information for public health has long been recognized. The

---

* Hetzel, A. (1997). *History and Organization of the Vital Statistics System*. Publication no. (PHS) 97-1003. Hyattsville, MD: Department of Health and Human Services.
† O'Carroll et al. (2003). *Public Health Informatics and Information Systems*. New York: Springer.
‡ CDC Healthcare Information Management Systems Society. (2012). CDC connecting to healthcare through interoperability. Retrieved from: http://www.cdc.gov/nchs/data/dvs/evital/14-CDC-HIMSS-2012-Interoperability-White-Paper.pdf.
§ MacDorman, M., and Kirmeyer, S. (2009). *The Challenge of Fetal Mortality*. NCHS Data Brief no. 16. Hyattsville, MD: National Center for Health Statistics.
¶ O'Carroll et al. (2003). *Public Health Informatics and Information Systems*. New York: Springer.

NVSS is viewed as "a source of credible national vital and health statistics for use by all levels of government, institutions and the general public."* Records of births and death provide the information needed for epidemiological investigations and surveillance. Information collected on the birth certificate includes such topics as teenage and unmarried childbearing, birth weight, length of gestation, smoking during pregnancy, access to prenatal care, and complications of labor and delivery.[†] Information collected on the death certificate includes the cause and place of death. The information obtained from vital records is used to monitor and understand trends in vital events and disease burden and to shape public health policies and investments.[‡]

Though NCHS does not have authority over the collection of vital registration data, the center engages in collaborative efforts, through the VSCP, to set standards and procedures for the uniform collection of information so that comparable data from all states can be combined to create national statistics. The National Association for Public Health Statistics and Information Systems (NAPHSIS), a national nonprofit organization that represents state vital records offices, facilitates interstate exchanges of ideas, methods, and technology for the registration of events and works with NCHS to promote uniformity among state systems.[§]

Two primary standards developed to promote the uniformity of data collection are the Model State Vital Statistics Act and the US Standard Certificates and Reports.[¶] The Standard Certificates and Reports are used to meet the legal needs of citizens and to record the information needed for public health purposes. These certificates are updated periodically with broad input from an array of stakeholders.** The current revisions are the 2003 US Standard Certificate of Live Birth (Figures 7.1 and 7.2), the 2003 US Standard Report of Fetal Death (Figures 7.3 and 7.4), and the 2003 US Standard Certificate of Death (Figure 7.5). Although these revised certificates and reports are in paper format, they were created as a standard data

---

* Hetzel, A. (1997). *History and Organization of the Vital Statistics System.* Publication no. (PHS) 97-1003. Hyattsville, MD: Department of Health and Human Services.

† O'Carroll et al. (2003). *Public Health Informatics and Information Systems.* New York: Springer.

‡ Nature Publishing Group. (2013). This week: Vital statistics. *Nature* 494, p. 281.

§ O'Carroll et al. (2003). *Public Health Informatics and Information Systems.* New York: Springer.

¶ Hetzel, A. (1997). *History and Organization of the Vital Statistics System.* Publication no. (PHS) 97-1003. Hyattsville, MD: Department of Health and Human Services.

**Centers for Disease Control and Prevention. (2012). National Vital Statistics System: 2003 revisions of the U.S. Standard Certificates of Live Birth and Death and the Fetal Death Report. Retrieved from: http://www.cdc.gov/nchs/nvss/vital_certificate_revisions.htm.

US Standard Certificate of Live Birth

Local file no.

Birth number:

Child	1. Child's name (first, middle, last, suffix)		2. Time of birth (24 hr)	3. Sex	4. Date of birth (mo/day/yr)
	5. Facility name (if not instruction, give street and number)		6. City, town, or location of birth		7. County of birth

Mother	8a. Mother's current legal name (first, middle, last, suffix)		8b. Date of birth (mo/day/yr)
	8c. Mother's name prior to first marriage (first, middle, last, suffix)		8d. Birthplace (state, territory, or foreign country)
	9a. Residence of mother-state	9b. County	9c. City, town, or location
	9d. Street and number	9e. Apt. no. / 9f. Zip code	9g. Inside city limits: ☐ Yes ☐ No

Father certifier	10a. Father's current legal name (first, middle, last, suffix)	10b. Date of birth (mo/day/yr)	10c. Birthplace(state, territory, or foreign country)
	11. Certifier's name: _____ Tittle ☐ MD ☐ DO ☐ Hospital admin. ☐ CNM/CM ☐ Other midwife ☐ Other (specify) _____	12. Date certified ___/___/_____ MM DD yyyy	13. Date filed by registrar ___/___/_____ MM DD yyyy

Information for administrative use

Mother	14. Mother's mailing address: 9 same as residence, or. State: ___ Street and number.		city, town, or location: ___ Apartment No:		Zip code:
	15. Mother's married: (at birth, conception, or anytime between) ☐ Yes ☐ No if no, has paternity acknowledgment been signed in the hospital? ☐ Yes ☐ No	16. Social security number requested for child? ☐ Yes ☐ No			17. Facility ID,(NPI)
	18. Mother's social security nubmer:	19. Father's social security nubmer:			

Information medical and health purposes only

Mother	20. Mother's education (check the box that best describes the highest degree or level of school completed at the time of death. ☐ 8th grade or less ☐ 9th - 12th grade; no diploma ☐ high school graduate or ged completed ☐ some college credit, but no degree ☐ associate degree (e.g., aa, as) ☐ bachelor's degree (e.g., ba, ab, bs) ☐ master's degree (e.g., ma, ms, meng, med, msw, mba) ☐ doctorate (e.g., phd, edd) or professional degree (e.g., md, dds, dvm, llb, jd)	21. Mother of hispanic origin? (check the box that best describes whether the mother is spanish/hispanic/latino. check the "no" box if mother is not spanish/hispanic /latino.) ☐ No, not spanish/hispanic/latino ☐ Yes, mexican, mexican american, chicano ☐ Yes, puerto rican ☐ Yes, cuban ☐ Yes, other spanish/hispanic/latino (specify) ___	22. Mother's race (check one or more races to indicate what the decedent considered himself or herself to be) ☐ White ☐ Black or african american ☐ American indian or alaska native (name of the enrolled or principal tribe) ___ ☐ Asian indian ☐ Chinese ☐ Filipino ☐ Japanese ☐ Korean ☐ Vietnamese ☐ Other asian (specify)___ ☐ Native hawaiian ☐ Guamanian or chamorro ☐ Samoan ☐ Other pacific islander (specify)___ ☐ Other (specify)___
Father	20. Father's education (check the box that best describes the highest degree or level of school completed at the time of death. ☐ 8th grade or less ☐ 9th - 12th grade; no diploma ☐ high school graduate or ged completed ☐ some college credit, but no degree ☐ associate degree (e.g., aa, as) ☐ bachelor's degree (e.g., ba, ab, bs) ☐ master's degree (e.g., ma, ms, meng, med, msw, mba) ☐ doctorate (e.g., phd, edd) or professional degree (e.g., md, dds, dvm, llb, jd)	21. Father of hispanic origin? (check the box that best describes whether the mother is spanish/hispanic/latino. check the "no" box if mother is not spanish/hispanic /latino.) ☐ No, not spanish/hispanic/latino ☐ Yes, mexican, mexican american, chicano ☐ Yes, puerto rican ☐ Yes, cuban ☐ Yes, other spanish/hispanic/latino (specify) ___	22. Father's race (check one or more races to indicate what the decedent considered himself or herself to be) ☐ White ☐ Black or african american ☐ American indian or alaska native (name of the enrolled or principal tribe) ___ ☐ Asian indian ☐ Chinese ☐ Filipino ☐ Japanese ☐ Korean doctorate (e.g., phd, edd) or professional degree (e.g., md, dds, dvm, llb, jd) ☐ Vietnamese ☐ Other asian (specify)___ ☐ Native hawaiian ☐ Guamanian or chamorro ☐ Samoan ☐ Other pacific islander (specify)___ ☐ Other (specify)___

Mother's name | Mother's medical record no.

26. Place where birth occurred (check one) ☐ Hospital ☐ Freestanding birthing center ☐ Home birth: planned to deliver at home? 9 yes 9 no ☐ Clinic/doctor's office ☐ other(specify)___	27. Attendant's name, title, and NPI Name:___ NPI:___ Title: ☐ MD ☐ DO ☐ CNM/CM ☐ Other midwife ☐ Other (specify)___	28. Mother transferred for maternal medical or fetal indications for delivery? ☐ yes ☐ no If yes, enter name of facility mother Transferred from:

Rev. 11/2003

Figure 7.1 2003 Revision of the US Standard Certificate of Live Birth (page 1).

set in anticipation of data collection and processing in an electronic era.* Therefore, edit specifications and other technical information were also developed and are available. By January 2016, all states were expected to have adopted the 2003 revisions.†

* O'Carroll et al. (2003). *Public Health Informatics and Information Systems*. New York: Springer.
† National Center for Health Statistics. (2015, July). National Vital Statistics System improvements (NCHS fact sheet). Retrieved from: http://www.cdc.gov/nchs/data/factsheets/factsheet_nvss_improvements.pdf.

Mother	29a. Date of first prenatal care visit ___/___/___ mm dd yyyy ☐ no prenatal care	29b. Date of first prenatal care visit ___/___/___ mm dd yyyy	30. Total number of prenatal visits for this pregnancy _____ (if none, enter "0.")
	31. Mother's height _____ (feet/inches)	32. Mother's prepregnancy weight _____ (pounds)	33. Mother's weight at delivery _____ (pounds)	28. Did mother get wic food for herself during this pregnancy? ☐ yes ☐ no

Mother (continued)

35. Number of previous live births(do not include the child)	36. Number of other pregnancy outcomes (spontaneous or induced losses or ectopic pregnancies)	37. Cigarette smoking before and during pregnancy for each time period, enter either the number of cigarettes or the number of packs of cigarettes smoked. if none, enter "0."	38. Principal sources of payment for this delivery
35a. Now living 35b. Now dead Number _____ Number _____ ☐ None ☐None	36 a. Other Outcomes Number _____ ☐None	Average number of cigarettes or packs of cigarettes smoked per day. # of cigarettes # of packs Three months before pregnancy _____ or _____ First three months of pregnancy _____ or _____ Second three months of pregnancy _____ or _____ Third trimester of pregnancy _____ or _____	☐ Private insurance ☐ Medicaid ☐ Self-pay ☐ Other (specify)_____
35c. Date of last live birth ___/___ mm yyyy	36b. Date of last other pregnancy outcome ___/___ mm yyyy	39. Date last normal menses began ___/___/___ mm dd yyyy	40. Mother's medical record number

| Medical and health information | 41. Risk factors in this pregnancy (check all that apply): <br> diabetes
 ☐Prepregnancy (diagnosis prior to this pregnancy)
 ☐Gestational (diagnosis in this pregnancy)

 Hypertension
 ☐Prepregnancy (chronic)
 ☐Gestational (pih, preeclampsia)
 ☐Eclampsia

 ☐ Previous preterm birth

 ☐ Other previous poor pregnancy outcome (includes perinatal death, small-for-gestational age/intrauterine growth restricted birth)

 ☐ Pregnancy resulted from infertility treatment-if yes, check all that apply:
 ☐ Fertility-enhancing drugs, artificial insemination or intrauterine insemination
 ☐ Assisted reproductive technology (e.g., in vitro fertilization (ivf), gamete intrafallopian transfer (gift))

 ☐ Mother had a previous cesarean delivery <br> if yes, how many _____

 ☐ None of the above
 37. Infections present and/or treated during this pregnancy (check all that apply)

 ☐ Gonorrhea
 ☐ Syphilis
 ☐ Chlamydia
 ☐ hepatitis b
 ☐ hepatitis c
 ☐ none of the above | 43. Obstetric procedures (check all that apply)

 ☐ Cervical cerdage
 ☐ Tocolysis

 External cephalic version:
 ☐ Successful
 ☐ Failed
 ☐ None of the above

 44. Onset of labor (check all the apply)

 ☐ Premature rupture of the membranes (prolonged, 312hrs.)

 ☐ Precipitous labor (<3 hrs.)

 ☐ Prolonged labor (3 20 hrs.)

 ☐ None of the above

 45. Characteristics of labor and delivery (check all that apply)

 ☐ Induction of labor
 ☐ Augmentation of labor
 ☐ Non-vertex presentation
 ☐ Steroids (glucocorticoids) for fetal lung maturation received by the mother prior to delivery
 ☐ Antibiotics received by the mother during labor
 ☐ Clinical chorioamnionitis diagnosed during labor or material temperature ≥ 38°c (100.4°f)
 ☐ Moderate/heavy meconium staining of the amniotic fluid
 ☐ Fetal intolerance of labor such that one or more of the following actions was taken: in-utero resuscitative measures, further fetal assessment, or operative delivery
 ☐ Epidural or spinal anesthesia during labor
 ☐ None of the above | 46. Method of delivery

 A. Was delivery with forceps attempted but unsuccessful?
 ☐ yes ☐ no

 B. Was delivery with vacuum extraction attempted but unsuccessful?
 ☐ yes ☐ no

 C. Fetal presentation at birth
 ☐ Cephalic
 ☐ Breech
 ☐ Other

 D. Final route and method of delivery(check one)
 ☐ Vaginal/spontaneous
 ☐ Vaginal/forceps
 ☐ Vaginal/vacuum
 ☐ Cesarean
 If cesarean, was a trial of labor attempted?
 ☐ yes
 ☐ no

 47. MATERNAL MORBIDITY (Check all that apply) (Complications associated with labor and delivery)
 ☐ Maternal transfusion
 ☐ Third or fourth degree perineal laceration
 ☐ Ruptured uterus
 ☐ Unplanned hysterectomy
 ☐ Admission to intensive care unit
 ☐ Unplanned operating room procedure following delivery
 ☐ None of the above |

Newborn information

| Newborn | 48. Newborn medical record number

 49. Birthweight (grams preferred, specify unit)

 _____
 9 grams 9ib/oz

 50. Obstetric estimate of gestation:
 _____ (completed weeks)

 51. Apgar score:
 Score at 5 minutes:_____
 If 6 minute score is less than 8,
 Score at 10 minutes:_____

 52. Plurality- single, twin, triplet, etc.
 (Specify) _____
 53. If not single birth - born first, second, <br> third,etc.(specify) _____ | 54. Abnormal conditions of the newborn (check all that apply)

 ☐ Assisted ventilation required immediately following delivery

 ☐ Assisted ventilation required for more than six hours

 ☐ NICU admission

 ☐ Newborn given surfactant replacement therapy

 ☐ Antibiotics received by the newborn for suspected neonatal sepsis

 ☐ Seizure or serious neurologic dysfunction

 ☐ Significant birth injury (skeletal fracture(s), peripheral nerve injury, and/or soft tissue/solid organ hemorrhage which requires intervention)

 None of the above | 55. Congenital anomalies of the fetus (Check all that apply)
 ☐ Anencephaly
 ☐ Meningomyelocele/spina bifida
 ☐ Cyanotic congenital heart disease
 ☐ Congenital diaphragmatic hernia
 ☐ Omphalocele
 ☐ Gastroschisis
 ☐ Limb reduction defect (excluding congenital amputation and dwarfing syndromes)
 ☐ Cleft Lip with or without Cleft Palate
 ☐ Cleft Palate alone
 ☐ Down Syndrome
   ☐Karyotype confirmed
   ☐Karyotype pending
 ☐ Suspected chromosomal disorder
   ☐Karyotype confirmed
   ☐Karyotype pending
 ☐ Hypospadias
 ☐ None of the anomalies listed above |
| Mother's name   Mother's medical record No. | 56. Was infant transferred within 24 hours of delivery? 9 yes 9 no
 If yes, name of facility infant transferred
 To:_____ | 57. Is infant living at time of report?
 ☐ yes ☐ no ☐ infant transferred, status unknown | 58. Is the infant being breastfed at discharge?
 ☐ yes ☐ no |

Figure 7.2 2003 Revision of the US Standard Certificate of Live Birth (page 2).

Local file no.

US Standard Report of Fetal Death

State file number:

Mother

1. Name of fetus (optional-at the discretion of the parents) | 2. Time of delivery (24hr) | 3. sex (m/f/unk) | 4. Date of delivery (mo/day/yr)

5a. City, town, or location of delivery

5b. Zip code of delivery

6. County of delivery

7. Place where delivery occurred (check one)
☐ Hospital
☐ Freestanding birthing center
☐ Home delivery: planned to deliver at home? ☐ yes ☐ no
☐ Clinic/doctor's office
☐ Other (specify)_____

8. Facility name (if not institution, give street and number)

9. facility id. (npi)

10a. Mother's current legal name (first, middle, last, suffix) | 10b. Date of birth (mo/day/yr)

10c. Mother's name prior to first marriage (first, middle, last, suffix) | 10d. Birthplace (state, territory, or foreign country)

11a. Residence of mother-state | 11b. County | 11c. City, town, or location

11d. Street and number | 11e. Apt. no. | 11f. Zip code | 11g. Inside city limits? ☐ yes ☐ no

Father

12a. Father's current legal name (first, middle, last, suffix) | 12b. Date of birth (mo/day/yr) | 12c. Birthplace (state, territory, or foreign country)

Disposition

13. Method of disposition:
☐ Burial ☐ Cremation ☐ Hospital disposition ☐ Donation ☐ Removal from state ☐ Other (specify)_____

Attendant and registration information

14. Attendant's name, title, and NPI
Name: _____
Npi: _____
Title: ☐ md ☐ do ☐ cnm/cm ☐ other midwife
☐ Other (specify)_____

15. Name and title of person completing report
name _____
title _____

16. Date report completed
___/___/___ mm dd yyyy

17. Date received by registrar
___/___/___ mm dd yyyy

Cause of fetal death

18. Cause/conditions contributing to fetal death

18a. Initiating cause/condition
(Among the choices below, please select the one which most likely began the sequence of events resulting in the death of the fetus)

Maternal conditions/diseases (specify) _____

Complications of placenta, cord, or membranes
☐ Rupture of membranes prior to onset of labor
☐ Abruptio placenta
☐ Placental insufficiency
☐ Prolapsed cord
☐ Chorioamnionitis
☐ Other specify_____

Other obstetrical or pregnancy complications (specify) _____

Fetal anomaly (specify) _____

Fetal injury (specify) _____
Fetal infection (specify) _____
Other fetal conditions/disorders (specify) _____

☐ Unknown

18b. Other significant causes or conditions
(Select or specify all other conditions contributing to death in item 18b)

Maternal conditions/diseases (specify) _____

Complications of placenta, cord, or membranes
☐ Rupture of membranes prior to onset of labor
☐ Abruptio placenta
☐ Placental insufficiency
☐ Prolapsed cord
☐ Chorioamnionitis
☐ Other specify_____

Other obstetrical or pregnancy complications (specify) _____

Fetal anomaly (specify) _____

Fetal injury (specify) _____
Fetal infection (specify) _____
Other fetal conditions/disorders (specify) _____

☐ Unknown

18c. Weight of fetus (grams preferred, specify unit)
_____ ☐ grams ☐ lb/oz

18d. Obstetric estimate of gestation at delivery
_____ (completed weeks)

18e. Estimated time of fetal death
☐ Dead at time of first assessment, no labor ongoing
☐ Dead at time of first assessment, labor ongoing
☐ Died during labor, after first assessment
☐ Unknown time of fetal death

18f. Was an autopsy performed?
☐ yes ☐ no ☐ planned

18g. Was a histological placental examination performed?
☐ yes ☐ no ☐ planned

18h. Were autopsy or histological placental examination results used in determining the cause of fetal death? ☐ yes ☐ no

Mother's name _____
Mother's medical record no. _____

Rev. 11/2003

Figure 7.3   2003 Revision of the US Standard Report of Fetal Death (page 1).

| Mother | 19. Mother's education (check the box that best describes the highest degree or level of school completed at the time of delivery)
□ 8th grade or less
□ 9th – 12th grade, no diploma
□ High school graduate or ged completed
□ Some college credit but no degree
□ Associate degree (e.g., aa, as)
□ Bachelor's degree (e.g., ba, ab, bs)
□ Master's degree (e.g., ma, ms, meng, med, msw, mba)
□ Doctorate (e.g., phd, edd) or professional degree (e.g., md, dds, dvm, llb, jd) | 20. Mother of hispanic origin? (check the box that best describes whether the mother is spanish/hispanic/latina. check the "no" box if mother is not spanish/hispanic/latina)
□ No, not spanish/hispanic/latina
□ Yes, mexican, mexican american, chicana
□ Yes, puerto rican
□ Yes, cuban
□ Yes, other spanish/hispanic/latina
(specify)_____ | 21. Mother's race (check one or more races to indicate what the mother considers herself to be)
□ White
□ Black or african american
□ American indian or alaska native (name of the enrolled or principal tribe)_____
□ Asian Indian
□ Chinese
□ Filipino
□ Japanese
□ Korean
□ Vietnamese
□ Other asian (specify)_____
□ Native hawaiian
□ Guamanian or chamorro
□ Samoan
□ Other pacific islander (specify)_____
□ Other (specify)_____ |

| 22. Mother married? (at delivery, conception, or anytime between) □ yes □ no | 23a. Date of first prenatal care visit __/__/__ mm dd yyyy □ no prenatal care | 23b. Date of last prenatal care visit __/__/__ mm dd yyyy | 24. Total number of prenatal visits for this pregnancy _____ (if none, enter "0.") |

| 25. Mother's height _____ (feet/inches) | 26. Mother's prepregnancy weight _____ (pounds) | 27. Mother's weight at delivery _____ (pounds) | 28. Did mother get wic food for herself during this pregnancy? □ yes □ no |

| 29. Number of previous live births | | 30. Number of other pregnancy outcomes (spontaneous or induced losses or ectopic pregnancies) | 31. Cigarette smoking before and during pregnancy for each time period, enter either the number of cigarettes or the number of packs of cigarettes smoked. if none, enter "0." |

| 29a. Now living
number _____
□ none | 29b. Now dead
number _____
□ none | 30a. Other outcomes
number (do not include this fetus) _____
□ none | Average number of cigarettes or packs of cigarettes smoked per day. # of cigarettes / # of packs
Three months before pregnancy _____ or _____
First three months of pregnancy _____ or _____
Second three months of pregnancy _____ or _____
Third trimester of pregnancy _____ or _____ |

| 29c. Date of last live birth __/__ mm yyyy | 30b. Date of last other pregnancy outcome __/__ mm yyyy | 32. Date last normal menses began __/__/__ mm dd yyyy | 33. Plurality - single, twin, triplet, etc. (specify)_____ | 34. If not single birth-born first, second, third, etc. (specify)_____ |

| 35. Mother transferred for maternal medical or fetal indications for delivery? □ yes □ no
if yes, enter name of facility mother transferred from: _____ |

| Medical and health information | 36. Risk factors in this pregnancy (check all that apply)
Diabetes
□ Prepregnancy (diagnosis prior to this pregnancy)
□ Gestational (diagnosis in this pregnancy)
Hypertension
□ Prepregnancy (chronic)
□ Gestational (pih, preeclampsia)
□ Eclampsia
□ Previous preterm birth
□ Other previous poor pregnancy outcome (includes perinatal death, small-for-gestational age/ intrauterine growth restricted birth)
□ Pregnancy resulted from infertility treatment-if yes, check all that apply:
□ Fertility-enhancing drugs, artificial insemination or intrauterine insemination
□ Assisted reproductive technology (e.g., in vitro fertilization (ivf), gamete intrafallopian transfer (gift))
□ Mother had a previous cesarean delivery if yes, how many _____
□ None of the above | 37. Infections present and/or treated during this pregnancy (check all that apply)
□ Gonorrhea
□ Syphilis
□ Chlamydia
□ Listeria
□ Group b streptococcus
□ Cytomegalovirus
□ Parvovirus
□ Toxoplasmosis
□ None of the above
□ Other (specify)_____ |

| 38. Method of delivery
a. Was delivery with forceps attempted but unsuccessful? □ yes □ no
b. Was delivery with vacuum extraction attempted but unsuccessful? □ yes □ no
c. Fetal presentation at delivery
□ cephalic
□ breech
□ other
d. Final route and method of delivery (check one)
□ vaginal/spontaneous
□ vaginal/forceps
□ vaginal/vacuum
□ cesarean
if cesarean, was a trial of labor attempted?
□ yes
□ no
e. Hysterotomy/hysterectomy
□ yes □ no | 39. Maternal morbidity (check all that apply) (complications associated with labor and delivery)
□ Maternal transfusion
□ Third or fourth degree perineal laceration
□ Ruptured uterus
□ Unplanned hysterectomy
□ Admission to intensive care unit
□ Unplanned operating room procedure following delivery
□ None of the above | 40. Congenital anomalies of the fetus (check all that apply)
□ Anencephaly
□ Meningomyelocele/spina bifida
□ Cyanotic congenital heart disease
□ Congenital diaphragmatic hernia
□ Omphalocele
□ Gastroschisis
□ Limb reduction defect (excluding congenital amputation and dwarfing syndromes)
□ Cleft lip with or without cleft palate
□ Cleft palate alone
□ Down syndrome
 □ karyotype confirmed
 □ karyotype pending
□ Suspected chromosomal disorder
 □ karyotype confirmed
 □ karyotype pending
□ Hypospadias
□ None of the anomalies listed above |

rev. 11/2003

Note: This recommended standard fetal death report is the result of an extensive evaluation process. information on the process and resulting recommendations as well as plans for future activities is available on the internet at: http://www.cdc.gov/nchs/vital_certs_rev.htm.

Figure 7.4   2003 Revision of the US Standard Report of Fetal Death (page 2).

US Standard Certificate of Death

State file no.

1. Decedent's legal name (include aka's if any) (first, middle, last)		2. Sex	3. Social security number

4a. Age-last birthday (years)	4b. Under 1 year		4c. Under 1 day		5. Date of birth (mo/day/yr)	6. Birthplace (city and state or foreign country)
	Months	Days	Hours	Minutes		

7a. Residence-state	7b. County	7c. City or town

7d. Street and number	7e. Apt. no.	7f. Zip code	7g. Inside city limits? ☐ yes ☐ no

8. Ever in us armed forces? ☐ yes ☐ no	9. Marital status at time of death ☐ married ☐ married, but separated ☐ widowed ☐ divorced ☐ never married ☐ unknown	10. Surviving spouse's name (if wife, give name prior to first marriage)

11. Father's name (first, middle, last)	12. Mother's name prior to first marriage (first, middle, last)

13a. Informant's name	13b. Relationship to decedent	13c. Mailing address (street and number, city, state, zip code)

14. Place of death (check only one: see instructions)

If death occurred in a hospital: ☐ inpatient ☐ emergency room/outpatient ☐ Dead on arrival
If death occurred somewhere other than a hospital: ☐ Hospice facility ☐ Nursing home/long term care facility ☐ Decedent's home ☐ Other (specify)

15. Facility name (if not institution, give street & number)	16. City or town, state, and zip code	17. County of death

18. Method of disposition: ☐ Burial ☐ Cremation ☐ donation ☐ entombment ☐ removal from state ☐ other (specify):	19. Place of disposition (name of cemetery, crematory, other place)

20. Location-city, town, and state	21. Name and complete address of funeral facility

22. Signature of funeral service licensee or other agent	23. License number (of licensee)

Items 24-28 must be completed by person who pronounces or certifies death	24. Date pronounced dead (mo/day/yr)	25. time pronounced dead

26. Signature of person pronouncing death (only when applicable)	27. License number	28. Date signed (mo/day/yr)

29. Actual or presumed date of death (mo/day/yr) (spell month)	30. Actual or presumed time of death	31. Was medical examiner or coroner contacted? ☐ yes ☐ no

Cause of death (see instructions and examples)

	Approximate interval: onset to death
32. Part I. Enter the chain of events–diseases, injuries, or complications–that directly caused the death. do not enter terminal events such as cardiac arrest, respiratory arrest, or ventricular fibrillation without showing the etiology. do not abbreviate. enter only one cause on a line. add additional lines if necessary.	
Immediate cause (final disease or condition resulting in death) ⟶ a._____ due to (or as a consequence of):	____
Sequentially list conditions, if any, leading to the cause listed on line a. enter the underlying cause (disease or injury that initiated the events resulting in death) last	b._____ due to (or as a consequence of):	____
	c._____ due to (or as a consequence of):	____
	d._____	____

part II. Enter other significant conditions contributing to death but not resulting in the underlying cause given in part I	33. Was an autopsy performed? ☐ yes ☐ no
	34. Were autopsy findings available to complete the cause of death? ☐ yes ☐ no

35. Did tobacco use contribute to death? ☐ yes ☐ probably ☐ no ☐ unknown	36. If female: ☐ Not pregnant within past year ☐ Pregnant at time of death ☐ Not pregnant, but pregnant within 42 days of death ☐ Not pregnant, but pregnant 43 days to 1 year before death ☐ Unknown if pregnant within the past year	37. Manner of death ☐ Natural ☐ Homicide ☐ Accident ☐ Pending investigation ☐ Suicide ☐ Could not be determined

38. Date of injury (mo/day/yr) (spell month)	39. Time of injury	40. Place of injury (e.g., decedent's home; construction site; restaurant; wooded area)	41. injury at work? ☐ yes ☐ no

42. Location of injury: state: City or town:	
Street & number: Apartment no.: Zip code:	

43. Describe how injury occurred:	44. If transportation injury, specify: ☐ Driver/operator ☐ Passenger ☐ Pedestrian ☐ Other (specify)

45. Certifier (check only one):
☐ Certifying physician-to the best of my knowledge, death occurred due to the cause(s) and manner stated.
☐ Pronouncing & certifying physician-to the best of my knowledge, death occurred at the time, date, and place, and due to the cause(s) and manner stated.
☐ Medical examiner/coroner-on the basis of examination, and/or investigation, in my opinion, death occurred at the time, date, and place, and due to the cause(s) and manner stated.

Signature of certifier:_____

46. Name, address, and zip code of person completing cause of death (Item 32)

47. Title of certifier	48. License number	49. Date certified (mo/day/yr)	50. For registrar only - date filed (mo/day/yr)

51. Decedent's education-check the box that best describes the highest degree or level of school completed at the time of death. ☐ 8th grade or less ☐ 9th - 12th grade; no diploma ☐ High school graduate or ged completed ☐ Some college credit, but no degree ☐ Fssociate degree (e.g., aa, as) ☐ Bachelor's degree (e.g., ba, ab, bs) ☐ Master's degree (e.g., ma, ms, meng, med, msw, mba) ☐ Doctorate (e.g., phd, edd) or professional degree (e.g., md, dds, dvm, llb, jd)	52. Decedent of hispanic origin? check the box that best describes whether the decedent is spanish/hispanic/latino. check the "no" box if decedent is not spanish/hispanic/latino. ☐ No, not spanish/hispanic/latino ☐ Yes, mexican, mexican american, chicano ☐ Yes, puerto rican ☐ Yes, cuban ☐ Yes, other spanish/hispanic/latino (specify) _____	53. Decedent's race (check one or more races to indicate what the decedent considered himself or herself to be) ☐ White ☐ Black or african american ☐ American indian or alaska native (name of the enrolled or principal tribe) _____ ☐ Asian indian ☐ Chinese ☐ Filipino ☐ Japanese ☐ Korean ☐ Vietnamese ☐ Other asian (specify) _____ ☐ Native hawaiian ☐ Guamanian or chamorro ☐ Samoan ☐ Other pacific islander (specify) _____ ☐ Other (specify) _____

54. Decedent's usual occupation (indicate type of work done during most of working life. do not use retired.)

55. Kind of business/industry

rev. 11/2003

Figure 7.5   2003 Revision of the US Standard Certificate of Death.

Final 1/28/04

| Mother's medical record #_____ |
| For hospital use only |

Mother's name_____

Mother's Worksheet for Child's Birth Certificate

The information you provide below will be used to create your child's birth certificate. the birth certificate is a document that will be used for legal purposes to prove your child's age, citizenship and parentage. this document will be used by your child throughout his/her life. state laws provide protection against the unauthorized release of identifying information from the birth certificates to ensure the confidentiality of the parents and their child.

It is very important that you provide complete and accurate information to all of the questions. in addition to information used for legal purposes, other information from the birth certificate is used by health and medical researchers to study and improve the health of mothers and newborn infants. items such as parent's education, race, and smoking will be used for studies but will not appear on copies of the birth certificate issued to you or your child.

Please print clearly

1. What is your current legal name?

| First | Middle | Last | Suffix (jr, III, etc.) |

2. What will be your baby's legal name (as it should appear on the birth certificate)?

| First | Middle | Last | Suffix (jr, III, etc.) |

☐ Name not yet chosen

3. What do you usually live--that is--where is your household/resisdence located?

Complete number and street_____ Apartment Number: _____
(Do not enter rural route numbers)
City, town, or location: _____
County _____ State: _____
Zip code: _____ (or U.S. territiry, canadian province)
If not united states, *county*_____

☐ Yes
☐ No
☐ Don't know

Figure 7.6   Mother's Worksheet for Child's Birth Certificate (page 1).

In hospital settings, two separate worksheets are used to collect the information for the US Standard Certificate of Live Birth. The legal and demographic information is collected on the Mother's Worksheet for the Child's Birth Certificate (Figure 7.6), and the medical information is collected on the Facility Worksheet for the Live Birth Certificate (Figure 7.7).* Similar worksheets were developed for fetal death reporting. These worksheets were developed to encourage the collection of data from the best sources—in particular, that the medical and health information be gathered from the medical records.

---

* Centers for Disease Control and Prevention. (2012). National Vital Statistics System: 2003 revisions of the U.S. Standard Certificate of Live Birth and Death and Fetal Death Report. Retrieved from: http://www.cdc.gov/nchs/nvss/vital_certificate_revisions.htm.

Mother's medical record # _____
Mother's name _____

Final (2/5/04)

Facility Worksheet for the Live Birth Certificate

For pregnancies resulting in the births of two or more live-born infants, this worksheet should be completed for the 1st live born infant in the delivery.
for each subsequent live-born infant, complete the "attachment for multiple births." for any fetal loss in the pregnancy reportable under state
reporting requirements, complete the "facility worksheet for the fetal death report."
for detailed definitions, instructions, information on sources, and common key words and abbreviations please see "the guide to completing facility
worksheets for the certificate of live birth."

1. Facility name:*_____
   (If not institution, give street and number)

2. Facility I.D. (National Provider Identifier): _____

3. City, town or location of birth: _____

4. County of birth: _____

5. Place of birth:
   ❏   Hospital ☐
   ❏   Freestanding birthing center (freestanding birthing center is defined as one which has no direct physical connection with
       an operative delivery center.) ☐
   ❏   Home birth☐
           planned to deliver at home ❏ yes   ❏ no ☐
   ❏   Clinic/doctor's office ☐
   ❏   Other (specify, e.g., taxi cab, train, plane, etc.)_____ ☐

   *Facilities may wish to have pre-set responses (hard-copy and/or electronic) to questions 1-5 for births which occur at their
    institutions.

Prenatal

Sources: prenatal care records, mother's medical records, labor and delivery records

Information for the following items should come from the mother's prenatal care
records and from other medical reports in the mother's chart, as well as the infant's medical
record. if the mother's prenatal care record is not in her hospital chart, please contact her
prenatal care provider to obtain the record, or a copy of the prenatal care information.
preferred and acceptable sources are given before each section. please do not provide
information from sources other than those listed.

Figure 7.7   Facility Worksheet for the Live Birth Certificate (page 1).

Challenges with Current Data Collection Processes

The NVSS is a prime example of data collection and sharing between
national and state agencies that could reap huge benefits from the increased
use of information technology. Current provider practices of collecting data

on live birth, fetal death, and death events are mainly paper based.* Most hospitals and birthing centers utilize paper forms to capture the mother's/patient's information. Much of the medical information on births, fetal deaths and deaths is found in the medical record. For example, the birth information is typically reported by a clinician with knowledge of the labor and delivery on a paper facility worksheet which is then keyed into the states' electronic birth registration system (EBRS) by a birth information specialist (BIS). Alternatively, a BIS completes the paper facility worksheet by reviewing the hospital medical records and then keys the information into the EBRS.

The reporting of a fetal death is a combination of birth and death data. For hospitals that use an electronic fetal death registration system (EFDRS), the data are keyed into the EFDRS and submitted to the vital records office. A similar process is utilized in a death event, whereby information is entered into the state's electronic death registration system (EDRS).

These data are reviewed, queried, and edited by the state's vital records offices. Selected detailed data are then sent to NCHS for processing and dissemination, and to create multipurpose national statistics.[†] This data collection method is susceptible to data quality issues due to redundant data entry, and the potential for mis-/underreporting by both clinical and non-clinical hospital personnel.[‡]

Current data collection processes are also complex due to the multiple potential sources for the data. In hospitals and birthing centers, the medical and health information needed for the birth certificate and fetal death reports can be retrieved from different types of records—for example, prenatal care records, hospital fact sheets, labor and delivery logs, and newborn medical records. A similar process is carried out for the death certificate, with information coming from both the funeral director and the medical certifier (physician or medical examiner/coroner). Funeral directors retrieve the necessary information from the next of kin and the medical certifiers provide the causes and manner of death.

In their study of birth certificate data, Brumburg et al. concluded that the data could be potentially of greater utility if the accuracy and completeness

---

* O'Carroll et al. (2003). *Public Health Informatics and Information Systems.* New York: Springer.
† National Association for Public Health Statistics and Information Systems. (2013). More better faster: Strategies for improving the timeliness of vital statistics. Retrieved from: https://docs.wixstatic.com/ugd/b08966_83b7bfa9fef54335a0f0240061e984d5.pdf.
‡ Brumberg, H.I., Dozor, D., and Golombek, S.G. (2012). History of the birth certificate: From inception to the future of electronic data. *Journal of Perinatology,* 32, 407–411.

could be improved.* They suggest that data collection and entry using current methods is responsible for significant delays in data reporting and leads to the reduced utility of the data.† Although states now have electronic systems, significant improvements in efficiency and accuracy may be possible by interfacing with electronic health record systems (EHR-S) and with other systems such as newborn screening to automatically extract clinical data from the mother's EHR. Recent increases in the adoption of EHR-S have paved the way for such interoperability.

NCHS is working in collaboration with vital registration areas and NAPHSIS to test the feasibility of the electronic exchange of birth, fetal death, and death information between EHR-S and electronic vital registration systems (EVRS) to improve data accuracy, completeness, and timeliness. Ongoing collaborations and initiatives to enable interoperability between EHR-S and EVRS in an environment of increased technology and information management will be described later in this chapter.

E-Vital Standards Initiative

Within NCHS, there has been a growing interest over the past several years in the potential that EHR data might offer for the future of data collection and survey processes. Discussions were held within NCHS and with key stakeholders to focus on developing a strategy based on the hypothesis that data from EHR systems could be utilized for birth, fetal death, and death reporting, resulting in timelier, more accurate, and better quality data.‡ In 2007, the e-Vital Standards Initiative was launched to concentrate efforts to develop electronic health data standards to enable interoperable electronic data exchanges among EHR systems, US vital records systems, and potentially other public health information systems for birth, fetal death, and death events.§ To fulfill this goal, NCHS committed resources to develop a stan-

---

* Brumberg, H.I., Dozor, D., and Golombek, S.G. (2012). History of the birth certificate: From inception to the future of electronic data. *Journal of Perinatology*, 32, 407–411.
† Brumberg, H.I., Dozor, D., and Golombek, S.G. (2012). History of the birth certificate: From inception to the future of electronic data. *Journal of Perinatology*, 32, 407–411.
‡ Atkinson, D. (2012). Integrating the Healthcare Enterprise: Vital statistics and electronic medical records. Retrieved from: http://www.cdc.gov/nchs/data/dvs/evital/10-NAPHSIS-Vital-Statistics-and-EHRs.pdf.
§ Health Level Seven International. (2011). HL7 Version 3 Domain Analysis Model: Vital records, Release 1. Retrieved from: https://www.hl7.org/implement/standards/product_brief.cfm?product_id=69.

dards-based, uniform, and systematic approach for collecting and exchanging data for vital records purposes pertaining to birth, fetal death, and death reporting.

Discussions regarding the e-Vital Standards Initiative ensued with representatives from NCHS, NAPHSIS, and other vital records stakeholders. Concerns were expressed regarding the feasibility of using EHRs as a source of information for vital records reporting and whether the EHR approach for data collection would be beneficial to the vital records community. Several vital records stakeholders indicated that the probability of improving the timeliness, accuracy, and quality of vital records data, and the prospect of reducing redundant data entry utilizing the EHR approach would need to be tested and verified. Despite these debates and considerations, NCHS and the vital records stakeholders concluded that it was worthwhile to lay the foundation for standardizing the transmission of birth, fetal death, and death events as efforts toward developing and implementing EHRs were continuing. If NCHS had not been proactive in advancing the e-Vital Standards Initiative, the potential consequences might have been the development of systems by vendors for birth, fetal death, and death reporting that were not compliant with the 2003 revisions of the US Standard Certificate of Live Birth, the US Standard Certificate of Death, and the US Standard Report of Fetal Death. Another potential consequence was a delay in engaging the vital records community in the interoperability activities that were underway in other public health programs including immunization, early hearing detection and intervention, and cancer reporting.

In addition, in 2004, President G. W. Bush stated in his State of the Union address, "By computerizing health records, we can avoid dangerous medical mistakes, reduce costs, and improve care."* This served as the impetus for federal initiatives such as the establishment of the Office of the National Coordinator for Health Information Technology (ONC). It also established the goal for most Americans to have access to an interoperable EHR by 2014.

An issue of paramount concern that was expressed to NCHS by key stakeholders from state vital records offices focused on the type of data that would be acceptable to collect from EHRs for vital records data reporting. This led to the development of an NCHS position statement that would limit the scope of data specified in vital records electronic standards development activities. The position statement states:

---

* The White House. (2004). State of the Union address. Retrieved from: https://georgewbush-whitehouse.archives.gov/news/releases/2004/01/20040120-7.html.

At this time, the NCHS/Division of Vital Statistics would prefer to limit the scope to a subset of the vital records data items for the first iteration of the developing standards. The jurisdictions legally responsible for the registration of vital events must be assured that the data received from the EHR-S are accurate and of high quality. Also, it is paramount to ensure that the source of the data for each data item is consistent with the requirements as defined in the NCHS Edit Specifications. Therefore, our initial goal will be to monitor and assess the quality of the data that will be exchanged between electronic health record and vital records systems through the implementation of demonstration projects. The primary focus for the death certificate will be to provide the necessary information in the EHR to assist the certifier in accurately determining the cause of death. Future iteration of the standards may include additional data items as determined.*

Since 2007, NCHS has been actively engaged in supporting the development of electronic health data standards for vital records (birth, fetal death, and death certificates). As reflected in the position statement, standards development work has focused on the medical information collected on the facility worksheet for the birth certificate and fetal death report. Additionally, NCHS has provided resources to support trial implementation testing and state implementation activities. Figure 7.8 provides a timeline of vital records standards activities from 2007 to 2013. Although the timeline only reflects activities through 2013, NCHS has continued to support the evolution of the

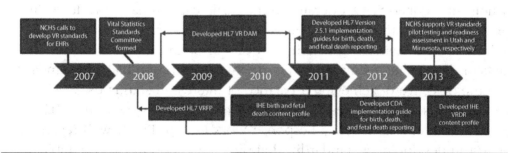

Figure 7.8   Vital records standards timeline 2007–2013.

---

* HL7 VRFP as Health Level Seven International. (2012). HL7 EHR-S Vital Records Functional Profile, Release 1---US Realm Chapter 1: Overview. Retrieved from: https://www.hl7.org/implement/standards/product_brief.cfm?product_id=17.

vital records standards with dedicated resources to remain actively engaged in work to support the e-Vital Standards Initiative.

Stakeholder Engagement

Identifying which stakeholders to engage in the e-Vital Standards Initiative was an important consideration for NCHS. State and jurisdictional vital registration agencies, SDOs, and EHR and vital record system vendors were identified as key vital records stakeholders to engage for this initiative. The state and jurisdictional vital registration agencies consist of vital registrars who would be responsible for providing subject matter expertise on the proposed vital records standards and would need to support any implementation activities. The role of SDOs would serve to provide a standards framework and a national, organizational structure for developing vital records standards. Vendor engagement was essential to support product development, trial implementation testing and implementation activities.

NAPHSIS was identified as a key stakeholder organization since it includes representatives from all states' and jurisdictions' vital records agencies. NAPHSIS formed an eHealth Committee that facilitated collaboration and discussion on the status of the vital records standards. NCHS solicited NAPHSIS members to reach out to the state and jurisdictional vital records offices to identify subject matter and technical experts to review and provide feedback on the draft vital records technical specifications throughout the standards development process and prior to publishing them as draft standards for trial use (DSTUs).

Health Level Seven International (HL7), an American National Standards Institute–accredited SDO, operates in the healthcare arena to produce clinical and administrative data standards for the healthcare domain.* HL7 utilizes a consensus-based balloting process to obtain feedback from participants of diverse interest groups who are interested in the balloted standards, with the objective of achieving a balance of interest in standards development activities. NCHS representatives presented an overview to the HL7 Public Health and Emergency Response Work Group (PHER WG) regarding interest in developing a standardized approach to support interoperability for exchanging vital records information. The work group recommended focusing on the HL7 Development Framework (HDF) and using its methodology

---

* Health Level Seven International. (n.d.). About HL7. Retrieved from: http://www.hl7.org/about/index.cfm?ref=nav.

as a resource to guide initial development work. The HDF is a "framework of modeling and administrative processes, policies, and deliverables that was developed by HL7 to produce specifications that are used by the healthcare information management community to overcome challenges and barriers to interoperability among computerized healthcare-related information systems."* These recommendations resulted in the development of the HL7 Vital Records Domain Analysis Model (VR DAM), which will be discussed later in this chapter.

During this time, a federal advisory body to the Secretary of the Department of Health and Human Services (DHHS) known as the American Health Information Community (AHIC) was chartered to make recommendations on how to accelerate the development and adoption of HIT. AHIC consisted of public and private sector leaders who represented a broad spectrum of healthcare stakeholders. They identified "breakthrough areas" in which the use of HIT could produce a tangible and specific value to the healthcare consumer that could be realized within a 2–3 year period. Population health and clinical care connections were identified as specific breakthrough areas for initial focus.

The Healthcare Information Technology Standards Panel (HITSP) was formed to serve as a multidisciplinary coordinating body charged with identifying the technical standards necessary to enable healthcare data interoperability and to promote standards harmonization for the breakthrough areas.[†] HITSP developed Interoperability Specification (IS) 91: Maternal and Child Health to describe the requirements needed to exchange obstetric and pediatric patient information between EHRs, including details to support the exchange of this information with appropriate public health programs.[‡] NCHS representatives participated in the HITSP activities, providing review and feedback on IS 91 during the public comment period to optimize consistency with the national requirements for vital records reporting. As the HITSP era ended in 2010, NCHS received recommendations from the HITSP Population Perspective Technical Committee to present IS 91 to Integrating the Healthcare Enterprise (IHE). The purpose was to suggest including the relevant requirements from the HITSP IS 91 specification in the IHE Maternal

---

* HL7 Development Framework. (2006). Retrieved from: http://wiki.hl7.org/index.php?title=HL7_Development_Framework.

† Healthcare Information Technology Standards Panel. (2009). About HITSP. Retrieved from: http://www.hitsp.org/about_hitsp.aspx.

‡ Health Level Seven International. (2012). HL7 EHR-S Vital Records Functional Profile, Release 1: US realm. Retrieved from: http://www.hl7.org/implement/standards/product_brief.cfm?product_id=17.

and Child Health trial implementation supplement. The HITSP specifications were incorporated as recommended in a subsequent publication of the supplement.

IHE is a standards-related organization that promotes the coordinated use of established standards to address specific clinical needs in support of optimal patient care by providing specifications, tools, and services for interoperability.* IHE creates detailed specifications, including content profiles, to describe specific solutions to integration problems by documenting how standards may be used to address interoperability problems.† As per the recommendations of the HITSP Population Perspective Technical Committee, NCHS representatives began to engage with IHE to learn about their products and to determine how they might support the development of vital records standards. The IHE Quality, Research, and Public Health (QRPH) domain had developed a Maternal and Child Health (MCH) content profile. The MCH was an overarching profile that consisted of two content profiles: the Health at Birth Summary (HBS) and the Child Growth Summary (CGS).‡

Initially, NCHS collaborated with the IHE QRPH members to provide feedback on the MCH profile. Later, NCHS decided to develop a new content profile that would specifically describe the EHR content that could be utilized and transmitted for birth and fetal death reporting for vital registration purposes. This led to the development of the IHE QRPH Birth and Fetal Death Reporting—Enhanced (BFDR-E) content profile that provided a key benefit of engaging with technical and subject matter experts including EHR and vital records vendors. NCHS also collaborated with IHE QRPH to create the IHE Vital Records Death Reporting (VRDR) content profile to support death reporting utilizing content from EHR systems. Additional details on the BFDR-E and VRDR profiles will be provided later in this chapter. Another benefit that NCHS gained through collaboration with IHE was the opportunity to engage in trial implementation activities with state agencies and key stakeholders from the EHR and vital records systems vendor communities.

---

* Integrating the Healthcare Enterprise. (2015). About IHE. Retrieved from: http://www.ihe.net/About_IHE.

† Integrating the Healthcare Enterprise. (2015). Profiles. Retrieved from: http://wiki.ihe.net/index.php?title=Profiles.

‡ Integrating the Healthcare Enterprise. (2009). IHE Quality, Research, and Public Health technical framework supplement: Mother and Child Health (MCH). Retrieved from: http://www.ihe.net/Technical_Framework/upload/IHE_QRPH_Mother_and_Child_Supplement_TI_2009-08-10.pdf.

HL7 Domain Analysis Model

Deciding where to begin with the standards development work at HL7 was a major consideration for the e-Vital Standards Initiative. Based on the guidance provided by the HL7 PHER WG, activities were initiated to develop an HL7 VR DAM. An HL7 technical contractor was secured to collaborate with representatives from NCHS, NAPHSIS, and other vital records stakeholders to provide detailed content for the model. An existing HL7 model, the HL7 Tuberculosis Surveillance, Diagnosis, Treatment and Research Domain Analysis Model, Release 1, served as a model and template for the VR DAM. The goal of the VR DAM was to publish a foundational standard that would identify the vital registration stakeholders, workflow processes, and vital records data exchanges while presenting the content in a format that would be understandable to both laymen and technical representatives.* The primary purpose for creating the model was to serve as a reference to guide future vital records standards design and implementation efforts and to lay the foundation for the standardized electronic transmission of birth, fetal death, and death events.

The HL7 VR DAM was published as an HL7 informative standard in April 2011. Storyboards, activities, and class models are included in the VR DAM. Vital records storyboards provide narrative descriptions to illustrate typical scenarios in which vital records information is collected and recorded on the 2003 revisions of the US Standard Certificate of Live Birth, US Standard Certificate of Death, and a US Standard Report of Fetal Death.† Activity models of typical birth, fetal death, and death processing in the United States are depicted utilizing flow diagrams to identify the workflow processes, stakeholders, and data exchanges that support data collection, record registration, and certified copy issuance.‡ The activity models in the VR DAM were developed to serve as a reference and resource on the workflow processes, stakeholders, and data exchanges specific to vital registration to guide the future development of the vital records interoperability specifications.

Figure 7.9 provides an example from the birth activity model. In this example, each column identifies a different entity that is involved in

---

* Health Level Seven International. (2011). HL7 Version 3 Domain Analysis Model: Vital Records, Release 1. Retrieved from: https://www.hl7.org/implement/standards/product_brief.cfm?product_id=69.
† Health Level Seven International. (2011). HL7 Version 3 Domain Analysis Model: Vital Records, Release 1. Retrieved from: https://www.hl7.org/implement/standards/product_brief.cfm?product_id=69.
‡ Health Level Seven International. (2011). HL7 Version 3 Domain Analysis Model: Vital Records, Release 1. Retrieved from: https://www.hl7.org/implement/standards/product_brief.cfm?product_id=69.

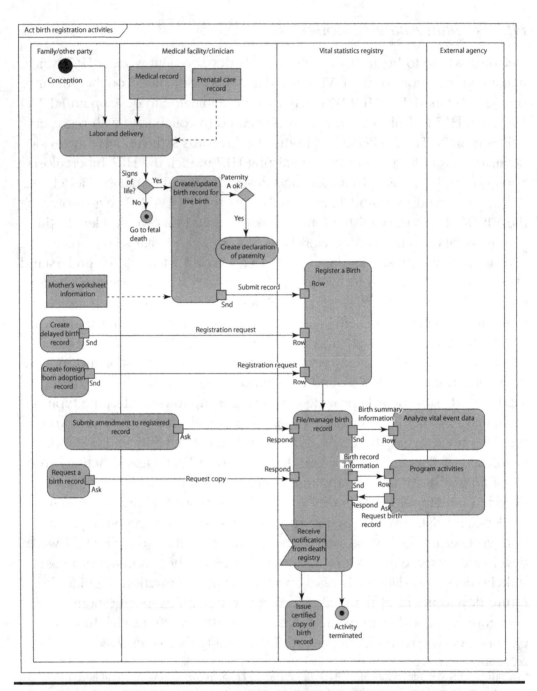

Figure 7.9 VR DAM birth activity model. (From Health Level Seven International, 2011. HL7 Version 3 Domain Analysis Model: Vital Records, Release 1, p. 13. Retrieved from: https://www.hl7.org/implement/standards/product_brief. cfm?product_id=69. With permission.)

activities surrounding a birth registration, beginning with the *Family/other party* and ending with the *External agency* that receives information about the birth. The dark circle identifies the beginning of the activities and the ending is denoted with a circle that includes a dot. The rectangular boxes represent documents that are utilized or exchanged during birth registration. The diamond shape indicates decision points throughout the birth registration activities that direct the flow of data and processes. Rounded boxes represent the various types of birth registration activities that are described in more detail within the VR DAM.

Birth, fetal death, and death class models illustrate the data that are captured for vital records purposes and the relationships among the data elements.* Class models were included in the VR DAM to serve as a reference and resource during the future development of the vital records interoperability specifications and to guide the identification of standard vocabulary for vital registration. A class death data model is shown in Figure 7.10. In the death data model, the boxes depict the data that are collected for death reporting. The data are aggregated and associated with a single data element. For example, all information or attributes collected about the decedent are included in the *decedent* class within this data model. The lines connecting the boxes show a relationship between some of the data that are collected. Numbers are included to show the cardinality or number of iterations that data may be collected for each data entry included. An asterisk suggests that more than one iteration may occur without placing limits on the maximum allowed.

HL7 Version 2.5.1 and CDA Vital Records Implementation Guides

Following the development of the VR DAM, there was a centralized focus on creating the HL7 technical specifications for transmitting medical information on births, fetal deaths, and deaths from a healthcare facility to a jurisdictional vital records electronic registration system. NCHS hosted teleconferences with vital records stakeholders to discuss and identify the type of HL7 standard to select for the technical specifications. After several presentations on the various types of standards and exploration as to the benefits of the various approaches, NCHS Division of Vital Statistics

---

* Health Level Seven International. (2011). HL7 Version 3 Domain Analysis Model: Vital Records, Release 1. Retrieved from: https://www.hl7.org/implement/standards/product_brief. cfm?product_id=69.

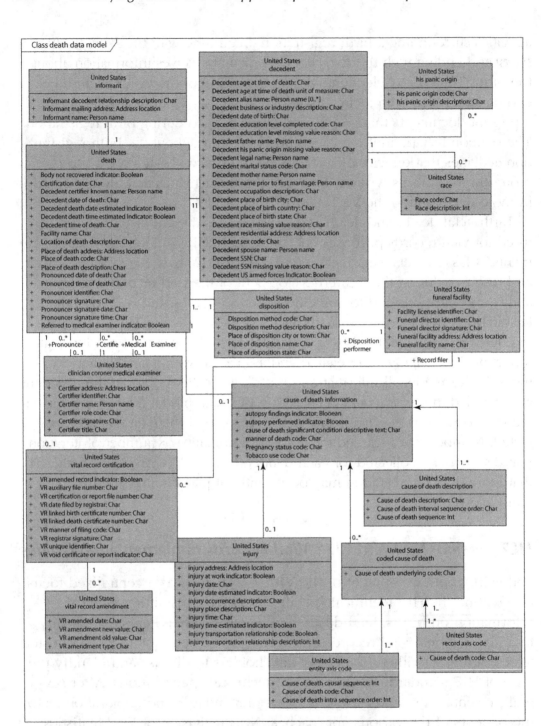

Figure 7.10 VR DAM death data model. (From Health Level Seven International, 2011. HL7 Version 3 Domain Analysis Model: Vital Records, Release 1, p. 58. Retrieved from: https://www.hl7.org/implement/standards/product_brief. cfm?product_id=69. With permission.)

Table 7.1 HL7 Vital Record Standards

Standard	Description
HL7 Version 2.6 Implementation Guide: Vital Records Birth and Fetal Death Reporting, Release 1—US Realm, STU	Provides a messaging implementation guide for transmitting birth- and fetal death-related information from a clinical setting to state vital statistics agencies and to the NCHS.
HL7 Implementation Guide for CDA Release 2: Birth and Fetal Death Reporting to Vital Records, Release 1 (US Realm)	Provides a CDA (document) specification for transmitting birth- and fetal death-related information from a clinical setting to state vital statistics agencies.
HL7 Version 2.6 Implementation Guide: Vital Records Death Reporting, Release 1—US Realm, STU.	Provides a messaging implementation guide for transmitting death-related information from a clinical setting to state vital statistics agencies, and to the NCHS.
HL7 CDA Release 2 Implementation Guide: Vital Records Death Reporting, Release 1 STU 2—US Realm	Provides a CDA (document) specification for transmitting death-related information from a clinical setting to state vital statistics agencies, and to the NCHS.

leadership decided to support the development of HL7 messaging specifications and Clinical Document Architecture (CDA). The decision was made to adopt the HL7 Version 2.5.1 messaging and CDA. This decision was based on the need for standard implementation options due to the variability in states' capacities. NCHS indicated that support would be provided to develop both types of HL7 standards for birth, fetal death, and death reporting.

Table 7.1 provides a list of the HL7 vital records standards that have been published as STUs.* HL7 members and other interested stakeholders can provide feedback on the STUs until the close date that is displayed on the comments web page. At the end of the comment period, NCHS plans to support the development of updated versions of the standards that incorporate the revisions as suggested via the STU comments and from feedback obtained from trial implementers. The goal will be to request approval to publish HL7 normative standards for each of the vital records specifications. Normative standards have been processed through the SDO and validated

---

* Each standard is posted on the HL7 DSTU comments website at: http://www.hl7.org/dstucomments.

with the intent to submit and obtain approval to publish them as American National Standards Institute (ANSI) standards.*

Although the HL7 vital records standards are currently STUs, they are already serving to help harmonize the development of new standards that include consistent or similar data content collected for vital records reporting. For example, in 2015, the HL7 PHER WG and the HL7 Structured Documents Work Group provided support for the development of an HL7 implementation guide for CDA Release 2 (CDA R2): Ambulatory Healthcare Provider Reporting to Birth Defects Registries, Release 1—US Realm. NCHS standards development participants and technical contractors provided comments on the birth defects standard and suggested revisions where appropriate for consistency with the vital records birth and fetal death reporting standards. This harmonization process is important to support interoperability across public health programs.

HL7 EHR-S Vital Records Functional Profile

NCHS involvement in HL7 also included participation with other industry leaders and organizational representatives in the Electronic Health Record Work Group (EHR WG) to develop the EHR-System Functional Model (EHR-S FM). The EHR-S FM offers a comprehensive set of functions and criteria that enable healthcare-specific applications to manage electronic healthcare information.[†] Functional profiles are then created as subsets to the model to support a standards-based method by which these functions and criteria can be applied to specific settings or domains.[‡]

In 2007, NCHS began work in collaboration with NAPHSIS and other industry stakeholders, including EHR and vital records vendors and healthcare providers, to develop the Vital Records Functional Profile (VRFP). The purpose of the VRFP was to identify the EHR system functions that support the capture of vital records information at the point of contact or point of care with the patient. The VRFP creates a common platform to describe the required EHR functionality for vital records. It also articulates

---

* Health Level Seven International. (2015). HL7 governance and operations manual. Retrieved from: http://www.hl7.org/documentcenter/public_temp_574CE5CD-1C23-BA17-0CEA28A6E571FBBA/membership/HL7_Governance_and_Operations_Manual.pdf.

† HL7 EHR-System Functional Model, R2. Retrieved from: http://www.hl7.org/implement/standards/product_brief.cfm?product_id=269.

‡ HL7 EHR-System Functional Model, R2. Retrieved from: http://www.hl7.org/implement/standards/product_brief.cfm?product_id=269.

the functional requirements needed to support messaging among providers, states, local registrars, and federal agencies.* An impetus for the creation of the VRFP was that it may serve as a source of reference for the certification of EHR systems that include functionality to better support vital registration. Additionally, it was intended to support the reduction of data errors by decreasing manual and duplicate entries of vital registration data, and thus improve data quality and the timeliness of data dissemination. Focus remained on medical information for births, fetal deaths, and deaths provided by the facility.

The creation of the VRFP necessitated broad input from stakeholders. Therefore, NCHS initiated a VRFP workgroup that included NAPHSIS members, NCHS subject matter experts, EHR and vital records system vendors, hospital and provider organizations, and related organizational representatives such as those from the American College of Obstetrics and Genecology and the American Pediatric Association. To ensure project success, NCHS formally engaged an expert appointee who was also an HL7 EHR WG co-chair with experience in developing the EHR-S FM and other functional profiles. He served to facilitate and provide expert technical guidance to the project. Additionally, NCHS funded the Public Health Data Standards Consortium (PHDSC) to provide logistical and communication support.

The VRFP project kicked off in June 2008 with a two-day workshop held at the NCHS headquarters in Hyattsville, Maryland. Participants were introduced to the structure of the EHR-S FM, then engaged in mapping the EHR system functions to the common use cases for birth and death and those activities that are common between the birth and death systems in the national Model Vital Events Registration System (MoVERS). A *use case* is a description of system behavior in terms of sequences of actions.† The descriptions presented in the use cases helped to identify the requirements of vital records present in the EHR-S FM. The edit specifications for the 2003 revisions of the US Standard Certificate of Live Birth, the US Standard Report of Fetal Death, and the US Standard Certificate of Death were also mapped to the EHR-S FM.

---

* Health Level Seven International. (2012). HL7 EHR-S Vital Records Functional Profile, Release 1: US Realm. Chapter 1: Overview. Retrieved from: http://www.hl7.org/implement/standards/product_brief.cfm?product_id=17.

† Health Level Seven International. (2012). HL7 EHR-S Vital Records Functional Profile, Release 1: US Realm. Chapter 1: Overview. Retrieved from: http://www.hl7.org/implement/standards/product_brief.cfm?product_id=17.

Subsequently, weekly calls were held to review each of the data elements identified on the national standard birth and death certificates, and fetal death report. They were compared to the functions and criteria contained in the EHR-S FM. The functional requirements in the model were then either accepted or modified to ensure adherence to the needs of vital registration, and new requirements were created as indicated. The project ended in 2011, resulting in VRFP documentation that describes a comprehensive set of functional requirements for the exchange of the medical information that could be collected in EHR systems and exchanged with vital records.

The VRFP was balloted through the HL7 ballot process and is currently an informative standard published on the HL7 website. Table 7.2 displays the structure of the VRFP and identifies the categories (i.e., Name, Statement, Description, and Conformance Criteria) that comprise a functional requirement. This particular table provides an example of the functional requirement for managing the newborn and fetal death information required for the US Standard Certificate of Live Birth and the Report of Fetal Death. The first column displays the function name and the second column provides a brief statement of the purpose of the function. The third column provides a more detailed description of the function, including examples if needed. The fourth column includes the sequencing for conformance criteria within a specific function. The fifth column outlines the conformance criteria that could be executed to perform the required function.

Following the development of the VRFP, NCHS partnered with other public health programs to expand the functional profile work to include additional domains within public health that may utilize similar functional requirements. This effort was aimed at supporting the harmonization of functional requirements across various public health programs. The result was the creation of the HL7 Public Health Functional Profile (PHFP), Release 1. The initial PHFP was balloted in 2011 (PHFP Phase 1) as an informative standard and covered three public health domains: namely, Vital Records (VR), Early Hearing Detection and Intervention (EHDI), and Chronic Disease (Cancer Surveillance).

In May 2013, an expanded version of the PHFP was balloted that included five additional public health domains: Public Health Laboratory Interactions (Orders/Reports) (PHLI); Health Statistics (HS); Occupational Disease, Injury, and Fatality (ODIF); Birth Defects (BD); and Deep Vein Thrombosis and Pulmonary Embolism (DVT/PE). The current version (PHFP Phase 3) contains a set of functional requirements identified for the eight public health domains from Phases 1 and 2, plus an Adverse Events health

Table 7.2   Sample from the HL7 Vital Records Functional Profile (VRFP)

R2 VR ID#	Type	N/A?	R2 VR Name	R2 VR Statement	R2 VR Description	C#	R2 VR Conformance Criteria
CP.3.3.2	F		Manage newborn and fetal death information required for the US Standard Certificate of Live Birth and Report of Fetal Death	Manage newborn and fetal death information required for the US Standard Certificate of Live Birth and Fetal Death	The phrase "newborn/fetal-death" is a term-of-art that identifies the subject-of-care who results from a "mother's/patient's" pregnancy. Newborn and fetal death information is documented on the facility and patient worksheets for vital records as specified in the NCHS/NAPHSIS ES. This information includes but is not limited to birth weight, obstetric estimate of gestation. Apgar scores, plurality, birth order, abnormal conditions, congenital anomalies, and facility transfers. It also indicates whether the infant is living at time of report and if the infant is being breastfed at discharge.	0	

(Continued)

Table 7.2 (Continued)   Sample from the HL7 Vital Records Functional Profile (VRFP)

R2 VR ID#	Type	N/A?	R2 VR Name	R2 VR Statement	R2 VR Description	C#	R2 VR Conformance Criteria
CP.3.3.2	C					1	The system SHALL provide the ability to capture all of the abnormal conditions and/or congenital anomalies of the newborn/fetal death as specified in the NCHS/NAPHSIS edit specifications (ES).
CP.3.3.2	C					2	The system SHALL provide the ability to render a report of all of the abnormal conditions and/or congenital anomalies of the newborn/fetal death as specified in the NCHS/NAPHSIS ES.
CP.3.3.2	C					3	IF the newborn/fetal death does not have any of the abnormal conditions and/or congenital anomalies specified in the NCHS/NAPHSIS ES, THEN the system SHALL provide the ability to capture a "None of the above" indicator accordingly.

Source: Health Level Seven International. (2011). HL7 Version 3 Domain Analysis Model: Vital records, Release 1. With permission. Retrieved from: https://www.hl7.org/implement/standards/product_brief.cfm?product_id=69.

domain. The PHFP was also updated to meet the new requirements and format of the HL7 EHR-System Functional Model, Release 2. Currently, the 2015 PHFP Release 2 is available for download from the HL7 website.

Vital Records Content Profiles

The HL7 vital records standards provide a standardized approach for transmitting and reporting birth, fetal death, and death information. The e-Vital Standards Initiative also emphasizes the potential benefits for abstracting information from EHR systems that is relevant for vital records reporting. IHE developed the IHE Information Technology Infrastructure (ITI) Technical Framework Supplement: Retrieve Form for Data Capture (RFD) Trial Implementation profile, which may be utilized for this purpose. The RFD profile supports the retrieval of forms from a form source, the display and completion of a form, and the return of data captured from the display application to the source application.*

RFD serves as the foundation for the two IHE profiles: BFDR-E and VRDR. These profiles provide support for data mining information that already resides within EHR systems that is relevant for birth, fetal death, and death reporting. For example, the BFDR-E profile provides a means to capture and communicate information from EHR systems that is needed to report births and fetal deaths for vital registration purposes. BFDR-E defines a specialized Labor and Delivery Summary for Vital Records (LDS-VR) document that may be used to prepopulate a *facility worksheet* form for collecting the medical and health information from an EHR for submission to a state vital records agency.† Implementers may provide functionality in their EHR systems that allows the birth information specialist to review, edit, and approve the completed facility worksheet information before submitting it to the state to report the birth event. Table 7.3 provides a description of the BFDR-E and VRDR profiles.

---

* Integrating the Healthcare Enterprise. (2017). IHE IT Infrastructure (ITI) Technical Framework Volume 1: (ITI TF-1) Integration Profiles. Retrieved from: http://www.ihe.net/uploadedFiles/Documents/ITI/IHE_ITI_TF_Vol1.pdf.
† Integrating the Healthcare Enterprise. (2017). IHE Quality, Research and Public Health Technical Framework Supplement Birth and Fetal Death Reporting—Enhanced. Retrieved from: https://www.ihe.net/uploadedFiles/Documents/QRPH/IHE_QRPH_Suppl_BFDR-E.pdf.

Table 7.3 IHE Vital Records Content Profiles

Content Profiles	Description
IHE Birth and Fetal Death Reporting-Enhanced (BFDR-E)	Defines the EHR content that may be used to prepopulate and transmit birth and fetal death information to vital records systems for vital registration purposes. Uses actors and transactions from the IHE ITI Technical Framework Supplement: Retrieve Form for Data Capture (RFD).
IHE Vital Records Death Reporting (VRDR)	Defines the EHR content that may be used to prepopulate and transmit death information to vital records systems for vital registration purposes. Uses actors and transactions from the IHE ITI Technical Framework Supplement: Retrieve Form for Data Capture (RFD).

Standardized Vocabulary for Vital Records

A well-structured vocabulary is essential for the collection and exchange of electronic information in a standardized format. When standardized vocabulary is used in conjunction with HL7 and related standards, it enables the exchange of clinical data and information by ensuring that sending and receiving systems have a shared, well defined, and unambiguous knowledge of the meaning of the data transferred.* SDOs such as the Logical Observation Identifiers Names and Codes (LOINC) and the Systematized Nomenclature of Medicine (SNOMED) promote the use of standard vocabularies to improve the interoperability of systems. NCHS has also adopted the use of standard vocabularies to enable and improve data exchange and interoperability between EHR systems and vital records systems.

The primary vocabulary systems utilized in the vital records standards are LOINC, SNOMED, and RxNorm. In 1999, LOINC was identified by HL7 as a preferred code set for laboratory test names in transactions between healthcare facilities, laboratories, laboratory testing devices, and public health authorities.† SNOMED provides a large, comprehensive computerized clinical terminology covering clinical data for diseases, clinical findings, and procedures.‡ RxNorm is a normalized naming system for generic and branded

---

* Health Level Seven International. (2012). Vocabulary: Charter. Retrieved from: http://www.hl7.org/Special/committees/Vocab/overview.cfm.
† Logical Observation Identifiers Names and Codes. (2010). LOINC and other standards. Retrieved from: http://loinc.org/faq/getting-started/loinc-and-other-standards.
‡ US National Library of Medicine. (2015). SNOMED clinical terms. Retrieved from: http://www.nlm.nih.gov/research/umls/Snomed/snomed_main.html.

drugs and a tool for supporting semantic interoperation between drug terminologies and pharmacy knowledge base systems.* NCHS promotes the use of these and other vocabulary systems to ensure consistent information for broad sharing and interoperability. Occasionally, the need for local codes still exists, and these are provided for through a CDC local coding system that is available to local, state, and national partners. The CDC coding system is termed the Public Health Information Network Vocabulary System (PHIN VS).[†]

The PHIN VS is hosted in the Public Health Information Network Vocabulary Access and Distribution System (PHIN VADS), maintained by the CDC. PHIN VADS is a web-based enterprise vocabulary system utilized to support public health and clinical care practice. It promotes the use of standards-based vocabulary to support the exchange of consistent information among public health partners.[‡] NCHS collaborates with the PHIN VADS team to include all vocabulary concepts that are used in the vital records standards. The repository also allows implementers to browse, search, and download the value sets associated with the implementation guides developed for the vital records standards. PHIN VADS presents views of the detailed vocabulary included in each of the vital records standards and is available from http://phinvads.cdc.gov, as depicted in Figure 7.11.[§] The view shown in Figure 7.11 lists each of the IHE and HL7 vital record standards. A viewer may see the list of vocabulary terms included in a specific standard by selecting the "Details" hyperlink. Further drilling down will provide an identification of the code for each item and the code system that is used.

In 2013, NCHS initiated the Vital Records Vocabulary Committee (VRVC) to support the development, review, and maintenance of vocabularies that will be relevant to the vital records standards. The VRVC includes representatives from NCHS, NAPHSIS, obstetricians and gynecologists, vocabulary specialists, and additional stakeholders and interested parties, as identified. Committee members collaborate on the selection, review, and maintenance of vocabulary standards to support birth, fetal death, and death specifications.

---

* US National Library of Medicine. (2015). What is RxNorm? Retrieved from: http://www.nlm.nih.gov/research/umls/rxnorm/overview.html.

[†] Centers for Disease Control and Prevention/Division of Health Informatics and Surveillance. (2015). PHIN vocabulary. Retrieved from: http://www.cdc.gov/phin/resources/vocabulary/index.html.

[‡] Centers for Disease Control and Prevention. (2015). PHIN Vocabulary Access and Distribution System (PHIN VADS). Retrieved from http://www.cdc.gov/phin/tools/PHINvads.

[§] Centers for Disease Control and Prevention. (n.d.). PHIN Vocabulary Access and Distribution Center. Retrieved from: http://phinvads.cdc.gov/vads/SearchHome.action.

View Name	Version #	
☐ HL7 V2.6 IG: VR Death Reporting STU R2 US Realm (Void Certificate)	1	Details
☐ HL7 V2.6 IG: VR Death Reporting STU R2 US Realm (Full Value Set)	2	Details
☐ HL7 V2.6 IG: VR Death Reporting STU R2 US Realm (NCHS->VR Coded R&E)	1	Details
☐ HL7 V2.6 IG: VR Death Reporting STU R2 US Realm (NCHS->VR Coded COD)	1	Details
☐ HL7 V2.6 IG: VR Death Reporting STU R2 US Realm (Null Certificate)	1	Details
☐ HL7 V2.6 IG: VR Death Reporting STU R2 US Realm (VR to NCHS)	1	Details
☐ HL7 V2.6 IG: VR Death Reporting STU R2 US Realm (Acknowledgement)	1	Details
☐ HL7 V2.6 IG: VR Death Reporting STU R2 US Realm (Provider to VR)	1	Details
☐ IHE QRPH Birth & Fetal Death Reporting - Enhanced (BFDR-E)	4	Details
☐ IHE Vital Records Death Reporting (VRDR)	2	Details
☐ HL7 Version 2.5.1 Implementation Guide: Birth & Fetal Death Reporting, R1 DSTU	3	Details
☐ HL7 Implementation Guide for CDA Release 2: Birth & Fetal Death Report, DSTU R1	2	Details
☐ HL7 Implementation Guide for CDA Release 2: Vital Records Death Report, DSTU R1	1	Details
☐ HL7 Version 2.5.1 Implementation Guide: Vital Records Death Reporting, DSTU R1	1	Details

Figure 7.11   PHIN VADS view of vital records standards.

Trial Implementation and Pilot Testing

Since 2011, NCHS has engaged with state agencies, provider organizations, and EHR and vital records system vendors to test the vital records standards. Each year, IHE hosts a "Connectathon," which is a structured testing event attended by hundreds of vendors, engineers, and architects from disparate vendor organizations. Participants test their products against multiple vendors using real-world clinical scenarios contained in IHE's profiles. Representatives from the Minnesota and Utah Departments of Health were funded by NCHS to enable their participation in the IHE Connectathon testing venues. Both states provided excellent feedback on the vital records standards as a result of their participation in the trial implementation activities. This resulted in additional standards development work with HL7 and IHE to refine, revise, and improve the technical specifications and content profiles in preparation for future testing and pilot implementations.

Additionally, trial implementation testing has led to the successful implementation of the HL7 Version 2.5.1 VRDR implementation guide by the Utah Department of Health in collaboration with Intermountain Healthcare, a healthcare system. NCHS provided funding support to facilitate testing and implementation activities for Utah to serve as a pilot state and provide a "proof of concept" for reference by other interested vital records stakeholders. The goal of this project is to strengthen the NVSS, improve the VSCP program at all levels, and facilitate the collection of appropriate data at the federal level.

Minnesota specifically engaged one of their state's provider organizations to participate in the IHE New Directions program, also known as the IHE Projectathon. The Projectathon provided an opportunity for stakeholder engagement with a specific organization to demonstrate a proof of concept and readiness for implementing the vital records standards.* Minnesota also received funding support from NCHS for a project to evaluate and determine their readiness for the adoption and use of the birth standards, and to make recommendations and identify next steps for implementation statewide.† Collaboration with provider organizations and state vital records agencies early in the standards development process has provided critical feedback to advance the e-Vital Standards Initiative.

Each year following the IHE Connectathon, state representatives and EHR and vital records system vendors have participated in the annual Healthcare Information and Management Systems Society (HIMSS) Interoperability Showcase. The HIMSS Interoperability Showcase features scenarios that depict unique events where healthcare stakeholders come together to demonstrate the benefits of using standards-based interoperable health IT solutions for effective and secure health data information exchange.‡ Vital records stakeholders have participated in demonstrations with other public health programs such as EHDI and Family Planning to illustrate interoperability for real-world scenarios using standard implementations.

As a result of trial implementation activities during the IHE Connectathons and the HIMSS demonstrations, the EHR vendor Epic decided to incorporate functionality within the Epic 2012 and later product releases to support electronic birth certificate submissions to state vital records agencies. The vital records system vendor, Genesis, has also provided support within their product line to interface the EBRS and the EDRS

---

* Integrating the Healthcare Enterprise. (2009). New directions process. Retrieved from: http://wiki.ihe.net/index.php/New_Directions_Process.

† Minnesota Department of Health. (2014). Minnesota e-Birth Records Project: Assessing readiness for e-birth records standards. Retrieved from: https://www.cdc.gov/nchs/data/dvs/evital/6-Minnesota-eBirth-Records.pdf.

‡ Integrating the Healthcare Enterprise. (2016). HIMSS interoperability showcase—A live demonstration of interoperability. Retrieved from: http://www.iheusa.org/ihe-demonstrations#Showcase.

with EHR systems. These products provide an opportunity for pilot implementation activities with provider organizations that have implemented
or plan to implement these products. NCHS continues efforts to outreach
to EHR and vital records system vendors to encourage participation in
trial implementation activities to further advance the development of the
vital records standards and to include functionality within their products
to facilitate broader outreach and implementation with provider and state
organizations.

Recently, NCHS has funded two projects to help advance the e-Vital
Standards Initiative. The first project will serve to evaluate the quality of
selected birth data extracted from EHR systems in two diverse vital records
jurisdictions compared with that reported on birth certificates for selected
maternal and child data elements for a retrospective sample of births. If
the project verifies the validity of the EHR extracted data, the selected
state health departments will have a methodology and metrics for the initial assessment and ongoing quality control of birth certificate information
received from EHRs. This project will ensure that, as the current manual
reporting process is replaced with automated reporting, the quality of data is
maintained or improved.

NCHS has also received Patient-Centered Outcomes Research (PCOR)
funding to support a project with a state to pilot the electronic exchange
of relevant death information between EHR systems and an EDRS using
nationally approved vital records standards. The project proposes to
improve the mortality data infrastructure for patient-centered outcomes
research by delivering state mortality records to the National Death Index
database in a more timely fashion through the more efficient data capture
of relevant death information from EHR systems. Improving the exchange
of death information will strengthen the NVSS as a whole and enhance the
VSCP at all levels.

Future Direction for E-Vital Standards

The current standards serve to enhance data collection and exchange
between EHR systems and vital registration systems utilizing national standards. However, states may collect additional data based on state and
jurisdictional laws. NCHS plans to embark on methods to standardize and
harmonize, where possible, these additional data elements so maximum
interoperability can be achieved.

Another future consideration is the transmission of standardized data from vital records offices to the federal agencies, particularly NCHS. Work is ongoing to extend the vital records standards to support interoperable data exchange between NCHS and state agencies. Further pilot testing and trial implementations will serve to identify errors and refine the standards to enhance the interoperability of systems, while assessing the business practices that may or may not need to change if electronic transfer is instituted.

Several projects are underway to increase the number of states and their capacity to participate in trial implementation activities. An outreach campaign has been started to inform all states and jurisdictions of the availability of the current standards and of the intent of NCHS to support and promote the use of the vital records standards. The NCHS website (http://www.cdc.gov/nchs/nvss/evital_standards_intiatives.htm) hosts current information regarding these initiatives and contains materials that states can utilize to inform other stakeholders to make the case for standards-based vital records interoperability.

Integral to the implementation of systems to facilitate the exchange of standardized information is the need for assurance that the particular system that is implemented will perform the necessary functions for which it is intended. Initially, NCHS has supported the Public Health Informatics Institute (PHII) to develop a report titled "Enhancing Electronic Health Record Systems to Generate and Exchange Data with Electronic Vital Registration Systems."* This report explores the possible roadmaps toward the potential certification of systems to ensure system capabilities. NCHS is considering recommendations and future strategies, which may include outreach to government-approved certification bodies to explore the potential for developing the certification criteria for vital records systems or, at minimum, assure conformity to the standards through conformity assessment programs.

The vision of interoperability faces several barriers to implementation. There are a limited number of EHR and vital records system vendors that have adopted and incorporated the vital records standards into their products since they are not recognized in the US Meaningful Use regulations.

---

* Friedman, D.J., and Parrish, R.G. (2015). Enhancing Electronic Health Record Systems to Generate and Exchange Data with Electronic Vital Registration Systems. Report prepared for the National Center for Health Statistics. Retrieved from: http://www.cdc.gov/nchs/data/dvs/evital/12-PHII-EHR-eVital-Records-Standards.pdf.

Currently, Epic is the only known EHR vendor that has incorporated functionality for vital records reporting into their EHR system products.

Conclusion

Efforts to improve the accuracy, completeness, and timeliness of vital events data collection have long been a priority of NCHS and the vital statistics program.* NCHS has supported the states in implementing the EBRS and the EDRS, and completing the implementation of the 2003 standard certificates and reports. As noted in the NCHS fact sheet on improvements to the NVSS, electronic birth and death records are expected to "improve timeliness of data, allow for transfer of data between states and integrate vital statistics with public health surveillance systems."† NCHS is also committed to activities and initiatives to test the feasibility of electronic data exchange between the EHR-S and EVRS.

The value of utilizing EHR data for vital records reporting has yet to be realized. At this point, NCHS believes the hypothesis that the timeliness, quality, and accuracy of data reported by providers to vital records agencies and ultimately to NCHS will improve. Based on this premise, NCHS has been and continues to be committed to supporting the development of standards and trial implementation activities. As pilot implementation efforts proceed and results can be analyzed, NCHS will assess the value of this standards-based approach using EHR data for vital records reporting. Providers, state agencies, and other vital records stakeholders will need to become more actively engaged in testing these standards if the vision of the e-Vital Standards Initiative are to be realized.

---

* Hetzel, A. (1997). *History and Organization of the Vital Statistics System.* Publication no. (PHS) 97-1003. Hyattsville, MA: Department of Health and Human Services.
† National Center for Health Statistics. (2015, July). Improvements to the National Vital Statistics System (NCHS fact sheet). Retrieved from: http://www.cdc.gov/nchs/data/factsheets/factsheet_nvss_improvements.pdf.

Chapter 8

Minnesota E-Birth Records Project: Assessing Readiness for E-Birth Records Standards

Kari Guida and Sally Almond

Contents

Introduction and Background

Minnesota, home to 68,783* births at 109 hospitals and freestanding birth centers in 2012, has long known the valuable resource that is vital records data and has worked consistently to engage its hospitals and birth centers in birth data improvement. Regular feedback to facilities, ongoing training and technical assistance, and an annual statewide training conference[†] has raised awareness of the importance of birth registration. Having improved the timely filing of birth records while reducing the number of unknown responses contained in those records, the Minnesota Department of Health's (MDH) Office of Vital Records is looking for ways to increase the quality and reliability of birth data without sacrificing timeliness. The state is also home to the Minnesota e-Health Initiative (the Initiative), which is legislatively chartered to coordinate and recommend e-health policies and priorities. The Initiative, established in 2004, helped make Minnesota an early forerunner in the adoption and use of health information technology in order to improve healthcare quality, increase patient safety, reduce healthcare costs, and improve public health.[‡] In addition, both MDH and the Initiative recognized that the continual adoption of electronic health record (EHR) systems and the focus on the electronic exchange of health information for the Medicare and Medicaid EHR Incentive Programs create new opportunities and challenges for public health programs, including vital records. Understanding these activities and their impact on vital records is critical to the health of the population and the efficiency and effectiveness of public health programs. The National Association of

---

* MDH. Minnesota Center for Health Statistics. Health statistics portal: Birth queries. https://pqc. health.state.mn.us/mhsq/frontPage.jsp (accessed October 28, 2015).

† MDH. Office of Vital Records. Birth registration information. http://www.health.state.mn.us/divs/ chs/osr/birthreg/index.html (accessed October 28, 2015).

‡ MDH. Minnesota e-Health Initiative report to the Minnesota Legislature 2015. March 2015. http:// www.health.state.mn.us/e-health/legrpt2015.pdf (accessed October 14, 2015).

Public Health Statistics and Information Systems (NAPHSIS) documented that vital records programs are limited in their ability to prepare for and address the challenges and opportunities due to the lack of or limited financial, political, and human capital.*

These activities collectively and separately exhibited Minnesota's willingness and ability to develop and implement the Minnesota E-Birth Records Project to increase the quality and timeliness of birth records information. The National Center for Health Statistics (NCHS) provided funding and technical assistance to MDH to evaluate the readiness for the adoption and use of e-birth records standards and make recommendations for the advancement of the standards-based exchange of birth records information. The project focused on two standards:

1. The Integrating the Healthcare Enterprise (IHE) Birth and Fetal Death Reporting (BFDR) Profile, which describes the content used to prepopulate the facility's worksheet form that is used to generate a birth record or fetal death report with clinical information from the EHR. The profile describes the content used in automating the data captured for vital records purposes for the 2003 revisions of the US Standard Certificate of Live Birth and the US Standard Report of Fetal Death.
2. The HL7 Version 2.5.1 Implementation Guide: Birth and Fetal Death Information Reporting, Release 1 (US Realm), which is an initial effort to provide guidance and messaging infrastructure for transmitting medical/health information on live births and fetal deaths from a birthing facility setting to a jurisdictional vital records electronic registration system.

Although the e-birth records content and messaging standards are for birth and fetal death, this project focused only on the standards for the US Standard Certificate of Live Birth. Similarly, the 750 Minnesota home births (2012 data), which are filed on paper, were deemed out of scope for this project.

Methods

Minnesota utilized a collaborative, multipronged approach during the project duration of September 2012–April 2014.

---

* NAPHSIS. More better faster: Strategies for improving the timeliness of vital statistics. April 2013.

Collaborative Team Model

Recognizing the variable resources available, MDH used a participatory collaborative project team model to utilize input from multiple disciplines, comprising staff from the state IT department and the Offices of Vital Records and Health Information Technology, found within MDH's Division of Health Policy. The team included a project manager, business/program experts, information technology experts, health informaticians, and project sponsors.

Stakeholder Engagement

This project team worked with the Minnesota Hospital Association to communicate and identify participation from Minnesota hospitals. Because interest in health information exchange expands beyond birth registration, all Minnesota hospitals (148) and independent birthing centers (4) were recruited via conventional letters and email in the fall of 2012. Hospitals and individuals were invited to participate in three areas: (1) community of interest, (2) advisory group membership, and (3) willingness to be a partner hospital or health system.

The *community of interest* was open to organizations or individuals interested in vital records and the standards-based exchange of health information. Invitations were extended to hospitals and birth centers, along with public health, vital records, and e-health experts. Periodic communications updated, educated, and engaged members of the community of interest in topics relating to the E-Birth Records Project, e-birth records standards, and e-health.

The *advisory group* met several times during the project. This group had a more direct impact on the project as members provided guidance, valuable insight to day-to-day operations, and limitations relative to birth registration, documentation requirements, and specific EHRs. Through in-person meetings and regular conference calls, the advisory group also recommended next steps and statewide policy. This 19-member group consisted of local, state, and federal experts in vital records, public health, and e-health, including representatives from six hospitals of varying size from separate, distinct Minnesota communities.

Two *local partners* had important and specific roles in the project.

■ Hospital A provided detailed data on current workflow, processes, and policies relating to collecting and submitting birth records. This hospital oversees more than 1000 births annually and uses an Epic EHR.

Table 8.1 Venues for Stakeholder Engagement

Minnesota	National
Annual birth registration conference and training (2013)	NAPHSIS/NCHS Conference (2013)
State e-Health Advisory Committee (2013–2014)	e-Health Initiative Conference (2013)
Department of Health leadership meetings (2013–2014)	American Medical Informatics Association (AMIA) Symposium (2013)
Annual e-health conference (2013)	Healthcare Information and Management Systems Society (HIMSS) Showcase (2013 and 2014)
Numerous internal and external meetings (2013–2014)	
State-coordinated response to Stage 3 definition of Meaningful Use of EHRs (2013)	

■ Health System Z provided the hospital and health system perspective on the technical readiness and needs of hospitals and collaborated to advance the e-birth record proof of concept at the 2014 IHE North American Connectathon. This health system uses an Epic EHR with Epic's additional Stork module, which is specifically designed for labor and delivery at its hospitals.

Throughout the project, stakeholder engagement and feedback was solicited through a variety of meetings, presentations, and events relative to vital records or health information exchange (Table 8.1).

Approach

The project focused on analyzing information, policy, workflow, and technology, and on testing the e-birth records standards.

Analyzing Information, Policy, Workflow, and Technology

The analysis of information, policy, workflow, and technology occurred primarily at the local (hospital) and state (MDH) level, along with some study at the national (NAPHSIS, NCHS) level.

Table 8.2 Testing and Showcasing Events

2013 IHE North American Connectathon
2013 HIMSS Interoperability Showcase
2013 NAPHSIS Interoperability Showcase
2014 IHE North American Connectathon
2014 IHE North American Projectathon
2014 HIMSS Interoperability Showcase

To fully understand and document the current birth registration process, *business process analysis* (BPA) was used at both the state office of vital records and Hospital A. Elements of the Collaborative Requirements Development Methodology from the Public Health Informatics Institute* were used to perform the analysis. The BPA consisted of a review of the processes, conditions, business requirements, and workflows surrounding the current collection and exchange of birth record information. This included identifying collected data elements, applicable policies, task sets, roles, timelines, and data usage. In addition, technology and data standards were reviewed. Data standards and collection tools identified during this process were analyzed for differences in content and structure. The findings were validated using local, state, and national partners involved in the advisory group, community of interest, and other stakeholder engagement activities.

Testing and Showcasing Standards-Based Exchange

Standards-based exchange was tested and showcased at five events (Table 8.2). Testing provides a proof of concept for the IHE BFDR Profile involving MDH, hospitals, and HIT vendors who tested systems' interoperability and conformance to the standards-based specifications in a controlled and monitored environment. These events convene to test standards-based information flow between separate and distinct partners in a test environment using the IHE BFDR Profile and the Retrieve Form for Data Capture (RFD) Profile.

---

* Public Health Informatics Institute. Collaborative Requirements Development Methodology (CRDM). Available at: http://phii.org/crdm (accessed December 24, 2013).

In addition, some of the events showcased the work of the project and partners. At the showcases, tours followed the flow of information from partner to partner. This provided the opportunity for education on the value of e-birth records and to build support for the e-birth records standards.

Findings

Birth Registration Process

A high-level view of the Minnesota birth registration process as identified by the project is illustrated in Figure 8.1. Birth record information is used by internal programs and organizations external to MDH. These programs use the information for public health surveillance and to target interventions. External organizations that use limited birth information include school districts, NCHS, other states and territories, the Minnesota Department of Human Services, the Social Security Administration, and local health departments. Although some of the inputs and outputs from the process were out of scope for the project, the sources and uses of birth data are necessary considerations for e-birth records standards development.

Minnesota Department of Health's Birth Registration Process

The BPA revealed internal and external users of birth data (Figure 8.1). The process of submitting birth records from hospitals to MDH is primarily through interactions of birth information specialists with the electronic birth registration system (EBRS), which is an integrated, web-based application for birth, death, and fetal death registration, secure vital records storage and maintenance, and certificate issuance. State and local issuance staff members, hospital birth information specialists, funeral directors, physicians, and medical examiners enter, maintain, or use birth and death data in the same system. Minnesota staff support and maintain the custom-built application.

Many steps are taken to prevent data entry errors and assure completeness and compliance with national standards. The steps include both manual and automated processes. The EBRS initially checks for duplicate birth records and warns the birth information specialist if a possible match is identified. Throughout the data entry process, the system prevents omitted data and requires the user to verify unknown or unlikely responses. Birth information specialists can return to birth records after filing to correct or

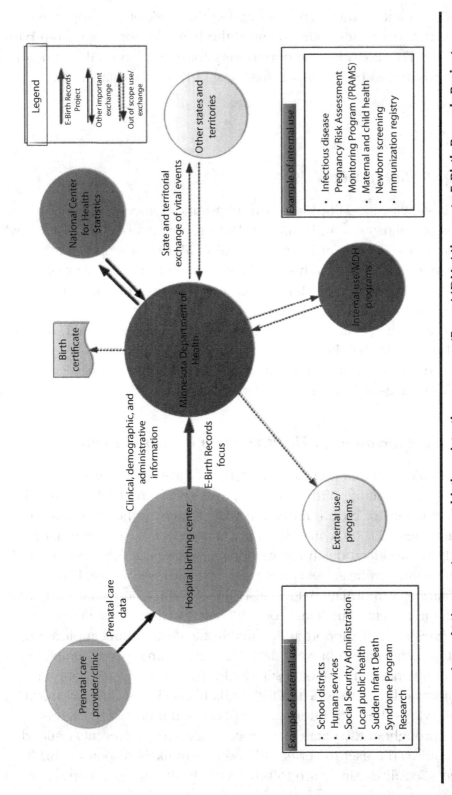

Figure 8.1 Overview of Minnesota's current birth registration process. (From MDH, Minnesota E-Birth Records Project: Assessing readiness for e-birth records standards, April 2014. http://www.health.state.mn.us/divs/chs/osr/birthreg/index.html, accessed October 15, 2015.)

add updated information. The EBRS prints verification forms for parents to view or proofread the data on their child's birth certificate. Staff at MDH offer training classes and telephone technical support to help birth information specialists enter complete and accurate birth records. Additionally, staff monitor "unknown" responses and will work with the hospitals to locate and correct health information that was not available during data entry.

Hospital A's Birth Registration Process

The hospital BPA focused on the birth registration workflow and processes to search, abstract, and submit birth registration information from Hospital A to the state health department. Similar to most Minnesota hospitals, Hospital A's process for birth registration is handled entirely by clerical hospital staff who complete 17 high-level steps during admission, labor and delivery, postpartum recovery, and discharge (Figure 8.2). Worksheets are given to parents to collect civil and demographic data for the birth record, and hospital unit coordinators acting as birth information specialists review patient medical records in the EHR to find applicable health information for birth registration. Many medical data elements present in the EHR are re-entered into the EBRS, including the mother's medical information, the newborn's medical information, and the newborn's initial assessment. The project team observed that a thorough review of the EHR is required to locate and report medical birth data and not all information is available as discrete data; some interpretation of narrative notes is required. When necessary, these staff members also help unmarried parents establish paternity for the birth record. These duties are in addition to other hospital functions and time constraints were noted. The hospital's process of collection, abstraction, and entry of information needed for one birth record could take less than an hour with no interruptions, or it could take several hours depending on competing duties, accessibility of information, and additional work activities and tasks.

Prenatal Care Data

Information about maternal prenatal care is an important part of the birth record; this information may be accessible at the hospital electronically or as a faxed paper document (Table 8.3). Associated prenatal care clinics utilize the same EHR system, so those patient's prenatal records are readily available electronically at Hospital A. Other prenatal care clinics routinely

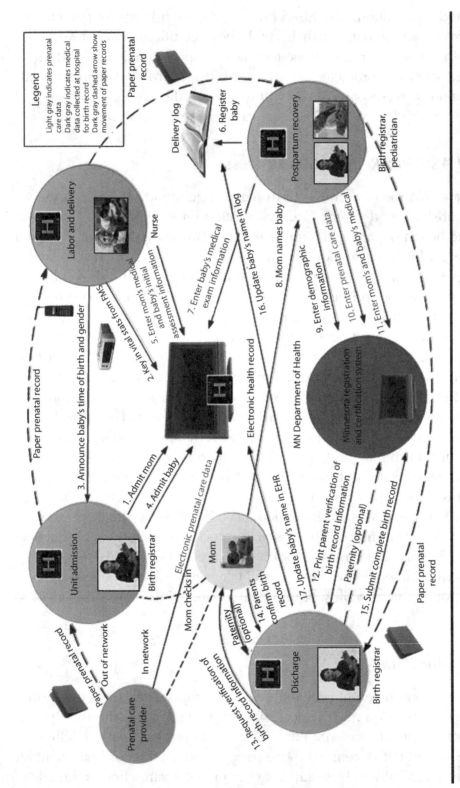

Figure 8.2 Hospital A's current birth registration process. (From MDH, Minnesota E-Birth Records Project: Assessing readiness for e-birth records standards, April 2014. http://www.health.state.mn.us/divs/chs/osr/birthreg/index.html, accessed October 15, 2015.)

Table 8.3   Sources of Prenatal Care for Hospital A

Source of Prenatal Care	EHR System	Format	Availability
Clinic affiliated with same healthcare system	Same EHR	Electronic	Through the EHR at time of admission at birth center and throughout patient stay
Associated clinic	Different or no EHR	Paper, faxed	Received at 36 weeks of gestation, prior to admission
No relationship to hospital	Different or no EHR	Paper, faxed	Requested from provider after patient admission at birth center

fax medical records for patients who plan to deliver at Hospital A when the patient reaches 36 weeks of gestation. Occasionally, this information is not received from the clinic prior to the patient's hospital admission for delivery, and hospital staff must contact the clinic to request the information. Table 8.3 shows the different sources for prenatal care data, their format, and whether it is accessible through the EHR. At Hospital A, if the prenatal care document is faxed, it will be available during the patient's stay in a special paper chart until discharge. These paper prenatal care data are not entered into the EHR's discrete or text fields at this hospital; instead, the documents are scanned as images into the EHR postdischarge. Stakeholders affirm the multiple sources of prenatal care. Ownership of patient health information is an issue. Some hospital policies prevent information from outside clinics, such as prenatal care data, from being scanned or entered into their EHR.

Collection of Medical and Civil Information

Birth registration data include both medical and civil information (Table 8.4). The medical information in the EHR is updated throughout the mother's and newborn's stay at the birthing center. Birth registration data are compiled from the labor, delivery, and immediate postpartum records for the mother, the newborn assessment, as well as the prenatal care record. Searching for and abstracting information from the EHR involves reviewing multiple EHR screens for information in both discrete and text or narrative fields. The location of information within an EHR varies, dependent on hospital, birth, EHR vendor/product, and provider.

Table 8.4   Birth Registration Data

Medical Information	Civil Information
Prenatal care • Visit history • Previous pregnancies and outcomes • Risk factors • Infections • Obstetric procedures	Newborn's name Mother's information • Name • Place and date of birth • Race/ethnicity • Marital status • Educational attainment
Labor and delivery summary (mother and newborn) • Delivery method and characteristics • Maternal morbidity • Newborn weight • Gestation • Apgar score • Abnormal conditions • Congenital anomalies • Breastfeeding	Father's information • Paternity establishment (if applicable) • Name • Place and date of birth • Race/ethnicity • Educational attainment

Civil information is collected from the parents during the birth registration process and included in the birth record. Upon admission to Hospital A, the mother receives the mother's worksheet, which is used to collect the newborn's name as well as the names, dates and places of birth, addresses, education, and race/ethnicity of both parents. The birth information specialist collects the completed worksheet and uses it to enter data into the birth record. Additionally, paternity acknowledgment documents may be filed by unmarried parents, which will become part of the newborn's birth record.

Electronic Fetal Monitoring System

The electronic fetal monitoring system is a medical device to observe and record the baby's heart rate and the mother's contraction activity during labor. This information is monitored and used to determine fetal distress during labor. These data are included in the birth record. At Hospital A, there is little or no interface between the fetal monitoring system and the EHR, so staff manually enter relevant data into the EHR. At other hospitals, work has begun to better integrate monitoring systems with the EHR. Other

EHR systems have their own fetal monitoring modules, such as Epic's Stork module, but many facilities manually enter the information.

Delivery Log

Hospital A maintains a delivery logbook or *baby name book* to keep track of births occurring in their birth center. In this paper log, birth information specialists write the newborn's information under the mother's last name, with a letter or number designating the order of birth; for example: "Smith, Baby A." Maintaining a paper log is a common practice at Minnesota hospitals, although the in-hospital naming convention varies among facilities. The log is updated by the birth information specialist when the newborn is named and serves as a reminder for birth registration staff to update the information in the EHR to reflect the child's legal name.

Comparison of Data Standards and Collection Tools

NCHS and Minnesota have each created data standards and collection tools, electronic and paper, for use in collecting data for the birth registration process. These standards, tools, and the e-birth records standards (IHE BFDR Profile and HL7 Implementation Guide) were compared with the 58 questions in the US Standard Certificate for Live Birth (standard certificate). This comparison identified three primary types of differences (Table 8.5).

Interoperability and the Minnesota Department of Health

The Office of Vital Records and other public health programs at MDH are experiencing an increasing demand from healthcare providers to electronically exchange health information using national standards. This demand for interoperability is a result of meaningful use and other health transformation activities such as the Minnesota Interoperable EHR Mandate (Minnesota Statute §62J.495 [Electronic Health Record Technology]). This mandate states, "By January 1, 2015, all hospitals and health care providers must have in place an interoperable electronic health records system within their hospital system or clinical practice setting." The mandate has led to high rates of EHR adoption in settings across Minnesota.*

---

* Minnesota e-Health Profile, MDH Office of Health IT, 2011–2015.

Table 8.5 Differences between Data Standards and Collection Tools

Type of Difference	Frequency	Explanation and Example
Standard certificate and e-birth records standards did not align.	22 of 58 questions on the standard certificate	1. E-birth records standards excludes civil registration data. For example, mother's education, race, and ethnicity excluded from e-birth records standards. 2. Standard certificate not updated to reflect recent NCHS and NAPHSIS policy decisions to eliminate some questions. For example: Was delivery with forceps attempted but unsuccessful? • Yes • No
Minnesota-specific responses for standards certificate questions.	27 of 58 questions on the standards certificate	Minnesota-specific responses were observed in additional options in value sets or differently structured date and time data fields. For example, principal source of payment for delivery question had Minnesota-specific responses of "Champus/Tricare," "Indian Health Services," and "Other government."
Minnesota-specific questions that were not on the standards certificate.	14 Minnesota-specific questions	Minnesota-specific questions were added to the birth registration. For example, mother's hepatitis B status and marriage status questions.

To meet this demand, an assessment of interoperability and health information exchange with a variety of public health programs with MDH is occurring. The focus is on MDH programs with applications accepting, using, and/or sharing individual-level clinical health information. The information learned from the assessment will be used to advance interoperability at MDH and to assure that resources are appropriated to meet the needs.

Testing and Showcasing Standards-Based Exchange

The testing achieved the goal of advancing the proof of concept and engaging new partners in the standards-based exchange of birth records. The technical mapping of data elements of the IHE BFDR Profile to Stork, an Epic Systems obstetric/labor and delivery product, was tested and showcased during the Connectathons, Projectathons, and Showcases. It should be noted that the testing only included the medical information of the birth registration process, which is part of the IHE BFDR Profile.

During the showcase tours and discussions with partners, numerous issues were raised that have implications or are related to readiness for e-birth records, including the following:

- The value that e-birth records standards could bring to public health, vital records, and hospitals is in the form of improved workflow, efficiencies, and the quality and timeliness of data. For example, more accurate and timely data could be used for quality improvement and measurement activities.
- Hospitals, EHR vendors, and states are currently focused on meeting the meaningful use requirements of the Medicare and Medicaid EHR Incentive Program. Without the inclusion of vital records as a public health reporting option or requirement, the adoption of e-birth records standards will be slow.
- The exclusion of civil information limits the value of e-birth records, as additional steps will be required to incorporate the civil information.
- Training and best practice recommendations will be needed to support and accelerate the adoption and use of e-birth records.
- Leadership from hospitals, state health departments, and vital records offices will be necessary for the adoption and use of e-birth records, but other priorities, including achieving Meaningful Use Stage 1 and 2, value-based purchasing, avoiding hospital readmission penalties, preparing for the transition to ICD-10, and various other health reform related activities, may hinder this support.
- The importance of the hospital's EHR vendor is significant as the IHE BFDR Profile is currently only mapped to the Epic Systems Stork module. The IHE BFDR Profile should be tested with additional EHR products.
- There has been minimal engagement by EBRS vendors in the development and testing of the e-birth records standards. In addition, the lack of standards for EBRSs has resulted in highly customized EBRSs for individual jurisdictions.

Discussion

The results suggest that MDH and Minnesota hospitals support the adoption of e-birth records standards but lack the readiness to fully test and implement them. The proposed Hospital Birth Registration Model (Figure 8.3) was developed to show the potential new birth registration process and information flow at a hospital if the birth records standards were adopted and in use. The proposed model has 9 high-level steps, compared with 17 in the current model. It utilizes the EHR as the source of information for the IHE BFDR Profile; all information about the mother and newborn would be available in the EHR and accessible to potentially improve future care events and outcomes. In addition, the proposed model engages the patient sooner and allows for multiple modes of communication between the patient and healthcare providers, increasing the convenience for both users.

The project identified key factors that will advance the readiness of hospitals and offices of vital records to adopt and implement the studied e-birth records standards across the nation.

Align Existing Data Standards and Tools

The line-by-line examination and comparison of current standards and resources revealed unexpected differences. Reducing or eliminating variations between national and state data collection tools and standards offer opportunities for improvement in both data alignment and the change management process. All vital records offices should fully explore and address any differences between the US Standard Certificate of Live Birth and the US Standard Report of Fetal Death and the state's information in preparation for the implementation of the e-birth records standards. Some state-specific data elements could be eliminated if found unnecessary or if other sources for data are identified. This comparison becomes a tool that, if kept up to date, can be used for change management, assisting in the identification, evaluation, and handling of changes to the birth records process and data standards and tools.

Build Offices of Vital Records' E-Birth Records Capacity

State vital records offices need to develop the capacity to support e-birth records. This capacity will need to include the training or retraining of staff, the development of policies and procedures, and engagement in

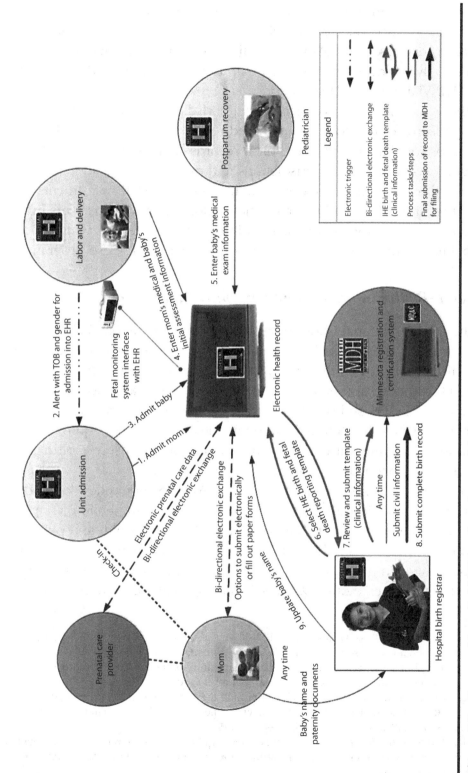

Figure 8.3   Proposed hospital birth registration model. (From MDH, Minnesota E-Birth Records Project: Assessing readiness for e-birth records standards, April 2014. http://www.health.state.mn.us/divs/chs/osr/birthreg/index.html, accessed October 15, 2015.)

agency-wide health information exchange planning. These capacity-building activities will advance vital records offices to informatics-savvy public health programs, as discussed by LaVenture et al.,[*] and support the adoption and use of not only e-birth records standards but other e-vital records standards such as IHE Vital Records Death Reporting.[†]

Another strategy to build capacity for all jurisdictions is for NAPHSIS and state vital records offices to develop shared requirements for EBRSs that align with or could align with the e-birth records standards. Not only does this create consistency across jurisdictions and prepare for the adoption and use of e-birth records, it could lessen the financial and staff investments from vital records offices to implement new information systems. This process has proven useful for immunization information systems,[‡] which is one of the public health programs that is part of the Meaningful Use program.

Advance E-Birth Records Interoperability Nationally

The Office of the National Coordinator for Health Information Technology (ONC) is working to increase interoperability and the use of standards on a broad scale. Although e-birth records have largely been untouched by the ONC, additional ONC and national activities can be leveraged to advance e-birth records. NCHS and partners should communicate about and develop guidelines to use the EBRS under the public health reporting requirements included in the Meaningful Use regulations and work to ensure e-birth records is part of nationally recognized standards.

National organizations such as NCHS and NAPHSIS should develop and implement a communications plan to show the value of and build community support for e-birth records. The plan should engage health and public health providers along with their associations and professional organizations. In addition, the plan needs to show the role e-birth records play in health reform, accountable care organizations, achieving health equity, improved

---

[*] LaVenture, M., Brand, B., Ross, D., and Baker, E. Building an informatics-savvy health department, part I: Vision and core strategies. *J Public Health Management Practice*. 2014;20(6), 667–669; LaVenture, M., Brand, B., Ross, D., and Baker, E. Building an informatics-savvy health department, part II: Operations and tactics. *J Public Health Management Practice*. 2014;00(00), 1–4.

[†] IHE. IHE quality, research and public health technical framework supplement: Vital Records Death Reporting (VRDR); Trial implementation. http://www.ihe.net/uploadedFiles/Documents/QRPH/ IHE_QRPH_Suppl_VRDR.pdf (accessed October 28, 2015).

[‡] Public Health Informatics Institute. Defining functional requirements for immunization information systems. 2012. http://www.phii.org/sites/default/files/resource/pdfs/IIS%20FINAL%2010302012.pdf (accessed October 28, 2015).

patient service, and improving population health. NAPHSIS and NCHS should incorporate e-birth records standards and e-vital records standards into the Vital Statistics Cooperative Program (VSCP)'s next five-year agreement.

Continue Expansion of E-Birth Records Standards

Although not ready for implementation, stakeholders can visualize the benefits of e-birth records standards. Prenatal care clinics are an important component to the process, yet they are deemed out of scope for the project. NCHS, NAPHSIS, hospitals, prenatal care providers, and state vital records offices should build support and demonstrate the need for antepartum profiles. This profile can facilitate the standards-based exchange of prenatal care information from the prenatal care provider to the hospital EHR as structured data.

Additional Considerations

The project identified numerous areas that were out of scope for the project but should be considered in future e-birth records standards work.

- It is generally believed that the implementation of e-birth records standards will improve the quality of the data. Additional research should occur to understand the relationship between e-birth records standards and the present quality of the data.
- Interoperability between EBRSs and other public health systems is another significant area of study to improve the use and value of birth records data.
- There is a need for standardization and general requirements for jurisdictions' EBRSs. This could be a strategy to share the costs of application development and maintenance. This is also a possible opportunity to leverage the ONC certification of EBRS vendors and products.
- This project focused on parts of the interoperability stack identified by the Standards and Interoperability Framework, but more work is needed to fully realize the needs and benefits of interoperability for the birth registration process, including prenatal care providers and NCHS.
- This project focused on birth records, but the implementation of e-birth records standards would have implications on the fetal death reports and death reports. These implications should be studied.

Epilogue

Since the completion of the Minnesota E-Birth Records Project, events have occurred that relate to the findings and key factors of readiness. The ONC has a new process that "will coordinate the identification, assessment, and determination of the 'best available' interoperability standards and implementation specifications for industry to use to fulfill specific clinical health IT interoperability needs."[*] The findings of this process will be compiled into the Interoperability Standards Advisory, which is scheduled to be released annually and will allow annual public comment. Through recent public comments, both NCHS and partners have recommended the addition of standards and implementation specifications that support e-public health standards, including vital records,[†] and resources for state health departments and partners to implement.[‡] The ONC process annually offers a venue for NCHS, NAPHSIS, and states to publicly support the adoption and use of e-birth records.

NCHS has funded two reports to document the progress and identify strategies for e-birth records standards and the health information exchange of vital records. The Public Health Informatics Institute report[§] interviewed over 40 experts, whose comments validate the Minnesota E-Birth Records Project. Most significant was that the goal should not be the adoption and use of the e-birth records standards and health information exchange, but the value gained in improved the quality and timeliness of data. In order to advance the exchange of birth records between EHRs and EBRSs, the authors identified six potential paths that can be selected, depending on criteria used by NCHS and partners.

---

[*] ONC. Interoperability standards advisory. September 12, 2015. https://www.healthit.gov/standards-advisory (accessed October 29, 2015).

[†] Centers for Disease Control and Prevention, NCHS. Readiness for e-birth records standards: Addendum to the Minnesota E-Birth Records Project: Assessing readiness for e-birth records standards. August 2015. http://www.health.state.mn.us/divs/chs/osr/birthreg/evitalsaddendumrpt.pdf (accessed October 29, 2015).

[‡] Minnesota e-Health Initiative. Minnesota e-Health Initiative statewide coordinated response to the 2015 interoperability standards advisory. May 1, 2015. http://www.health.state.mn.us/e-health/ehealthdocs/coordrespnsstndrsinterop2015acfinal.pdf (accessed October 29, 2015).

[§] Public Health Informatics Institute. Enhancing electronic health record systems to generate and exchange data with electronic vital registrations systems. http://www.ncvhs.hhs.gov/wp-content/uploads/2015/04/NCVHS_Friedman-Parrish_2015_eVitals.pdf (accessed June 30, 2015).

The addendum to the Minnesota E-Birth Records Project* documents the advances in the adoption and use of e-birth records standards. Progress was documented in that additional EHR vendors have tested or discussed the option to test the IHE BFDR Profile. Additional buy-in for the work was gained when the May 2015 National Committee on Vital Health Statistics included an e-vital records project demonstration. This activity led to a discussion on the opportunities of e-birth records standards. Finally, progress was noted in that Meaningful Use Stage 3 will have flexibility in public health reporting and clinical data registry reporting, which may lead to some entities designating vital records as an option for the public health criteria.

---

* Centers for Disease Control and Prevention, NCHS. Readiness for e-birth records standards: Addendum to the Minnesota E-Birth Records Project: Assessing readiness for e-birth records standards. August 2015. http://www.health.state.mn.us/divs/chs/osr/birthreg/evitalsaddendumrpt.pdf (accessed October 29, 2015).

Chapter 9

E-Death Records in Utah

Jeffrey Duncan

Contents

Background

When a person dies of natural causes in the United States, a physician is required to enter a cause of death on a death certificate that is then registered with the vital records office in the state where the death occurs. The information provided by the physician is used to tabulate national mortality statistics,[1] to establish leading causes of death,[2] for public health surveillance,[3] and for biomedical research.[4] The information is also used to inform public health policy and biomedical research.

Utah state law requires deaths to be certified by a physician within 72 hours of death. Final registration of the death certificate must occur after physician certification; it must be completed within 5 days of death and is

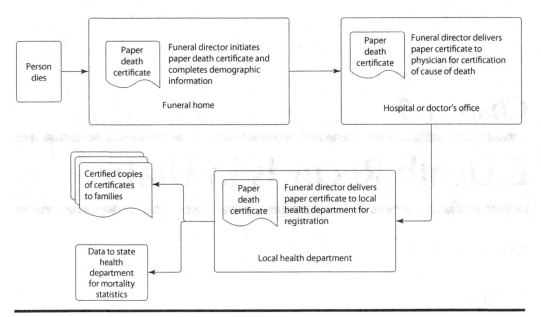

Figure 9.1 **Typical flow of paper death certificates.**

necessary before the funeral director may cremate or otherwise dispose of human remains (Utah Statute Title 26, Chapter 2).

Until the early 2000s, death certificates in the United States were entirely paper documents that were initiated by funeral directors following a person's death. The paper certificate was then delivered to a physician who was required to enter a cause of death and signature on the document. The completed document was then taken to a local health department official for registration and issuance. Figure 9.1 illustrates the typical flow of paper death certificates. With the advent of the Internet, many states began developing electronic death registration systems (EDRSs) to replace the time-consuming paper death certificate process. Typically, an EDRS provides a secure, web-based interface for all participants in the death certificate process (funeral directors, physicians, and state and local health department staff) to complete their portion of the death certificate electronically.

In 2006, the Office of Vital Records and Statistics (OVRS) in Utah implemented an EDRS known as the Electronic Death Entry Network (EDEN). EDEN was designed to replace the existing paper death certificate process with a web-based one that would enable physicians, funeral directors, and local and state public health personnel to interact and complete death certificates for deceased individuals. Figure 9.2 is an overview of the EDEN death certificate process.

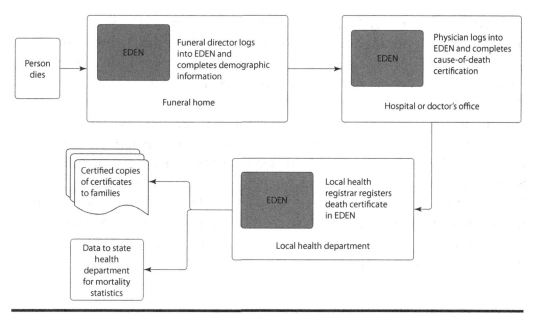

Figure 9.2   Typical EDEN death certificate flow.

While the flow of information in EDEN is similar to the paper process, the web-based interface allows all parties in the death registration process to complete their portions electronically. The EDEN system was well received by funeral directors because it eliminated the significant time and logistics of delivering a paper certificate for signatures to multiple locations. Within its first 3 months, 100% of all licensed Utah funeral directors were enrolled in and using EDEN to complete death certificates. Physicians, however, were not as eager to sign up for access to EDEN. The EDEN web application represented a new login and password to remember, and a new program to understand and use. As a result, typically only physicians who were in practice types such as end-of-life or acute care, with a concomitant need for frequent death registration, were willing to use EDEN for death registration. The remainder opted to use the slower, paper-based process.

In order to increase the percentage of physicians registering deaths electronically, in 2008, the Utah Department of Health (UDOH) applied for and was awarded a grant from the Centers for Disease Control and Prevention/ National Center for Health Statistics (CDC/NCHS) to implement an interface for physicians using Intermountain Healthcare's existing electronic health record (EHR) to certify death certificates. Interestingly, the idea was first proposed by an Intermountain physician who, while being trained on the EDEN system exclaimed to the author, "Why do I have to log in to your system? Why can't I just do the death certificate from my EHR?"

Intermountain, Utah's largest provider of healthcare services, was a likely place for death reporting from an EHR to begin, given that Intermountain serves over 50% of Utah's population and has been a pioneer in developing and using electronic medical records for over 40 years.[5] Intermountain's HELP2 system has been in operation for decades.[6,7]

The death certificate exchange between HELP2 and EDEN contains three major components: an EHR module that allows physicians to enter death certificate information into a familiar death certificate form, a Health Level Seven International (HL7) interface that allows data to be transmitted to UDOH, and a match-and-merge component at UDOH that merges physician-provided death certifications with funeral director–provided decedent information in EDEN. The following is a brief discussion of the development of each of these components.

Electronic Health Record Death Module

With the advent of EDRSs such as EDEN in the early 2000s, NCHS produced guidelines for the electronic capture of cause-of-death information. These guidelines were necessary to produce data consistency between death certificates completed on paper compared with those completed on computers. For the most part, these guidelines require online death certification forms to mimic paper forms in their format and textual instructions, and prohibit the use of things such as pick lists that may bias the selection of certain death causes over others. UDOH vital records staff worked with Intermountain software engineers to develop and test specifications for the EHR death module.

Another key component of the EHR component is the presence and functionality of field edits. Computer data entry screens allow for the use of processes known variously as *data validation, consistency checks,* or *field edits.* For example, if a value is entered for the date of injury, the computer can require other injury-related fields to also be completed before the form can be submitted.

Health Level Seven International Interface

In 2008, when work on the HL7 interface to carry death certificate information from Intermountain to UDOH began, there was not an existing standard message approved by the HL7 organization to carry such information. At the time, the only office within UDOH with significant experience developing HL7 interfaces was the Utah Statewide Immunization Information System (USIIS). USIIS technical staff worked with vital records subject matter experts and Intermountain interface engineers to agree on an HL7 message format that would meet the needs for death certification. The result was a message based on HL7's Admit, Discharge, Transfer (ADT) standard, using configurable Z-segments to contain death-specific information.

Match-and-Merge Component

In EDEN, the death certificate workflow nearly always begins with a funeral director creating a new record for a decedent. After completing demographic information, the funeral director notifies the certifying physician to log in to EDEN to complete the record. For non-EDEN users, a paper death certificate must be printed and delivered for the physician to complete by hand.

The implementation of the HELP2 interface complicates this workflow, as the physician and funeral director may now complete their parts of the death certificate asynchronously. A physician using HELP2 need not wait for a funeral director to initiate a death record in the EHR. Once completed, the cause-of-death certification is sent to UDOH over the HL7 interface. At UDOH, the information is parsed and stored in an EDEN table called *cause of death*. A match-and-merge process was developed to link physician-provided cause-of-death records with funeral director–provided demographic records in the EDEN database. Records are matched using demographic information that may be contained in both records, such as name, date of birth, sex, and social security number. Records must match in all respects in order for them to be automatically merged. If there is a discrepancy in name, for example, records will not merge automatically. Vital records staff periodically review a queue of pending records and manually force records to merge when there is not exact agreement in matching information.

In 2013, UDOH received funding from the CDC/NCHS to implement the HL7 V2.5.1 Implementation Guide: Vital Records Death Reporting, Release 1 Draft Standard for Trial Use (DSTU). The development of the DSTU is described earlier in this chapter. To implement the new standard, UDOH staff worked with Intermountain interface engineers to conduct a gap analysis and identify the extent of changes between the ad hoc HL7 message that was currently in production compared with the DSTU. The DSTU replaced local codes that were currently in use with standard value sets drawn from Logical Observation Identifiers Names and Codes (LOINC), Systematized

Nomenclature of Medicine (SNOMED), and the CDC's Public Health Information Network Vocabulary Access and Distribution System (PHIN VADS).

Methods

The initial implementations of HL7 messaging and the DSTU implementation both used transmission control protocol/Internet protocol (TCP/IP) over a virtual private network (VPN) as the method for transporting death messages from Intermountain to UDOH. At the time, VPN connections were standard practice for the Utah Statewide Immunization Information System (USIIS) and other UDOH external interfaces. The VPN transport method provides for the real-time exchange of information and excellent security and encryption, but those advantages come with significant challenges. Creating and maintaining an open VPN between two large enterprises such as a state government and a large healthcare organization requires careful coordination between network engineers at the facility and the enterprise level of each organization. Upgrades to network security or firewalls in either organization can result in closure of the VPN tunnel, requiring extensive troubleshooting to determine the cause when messages are not flowing properly.

In recent years, USIIS has begun using web service interfaces to securely transport HL7 messages, a growing practice in the healthcare industry. The web service approach is much easier to configure than a VPN, while providing the same real-time messaging capability.

Results

Technical Results

Since 2011, Utah has successfully improved the ability for physicians at Intermountain facilities to enter and certify deaths for their patients. The infrastructure created, including the interface engine and match-and-merge process, is available to provide this capacity to physicians in other healthcare organizations in Utah. To implement this capability, a healthcare organization would need to develop a data collection screen in its EHR and implement the HL7 V2.5.1 Vital Records Death Reporting messaging DSTU. To avoid repeated re-creation of the data collection form across different vendors' EHRs, UDOH is working with CDC to implement and test standards-based death reporting using the Integrating the Healthcare Enterprise (IHE) Retrieve Form for Data Capture (RFD) exchange profile.

Operational Results

We conducted a formal evaluation of cause-of-death information collected from the Intermountain EHR compared with death certificate information collected through EDEN or paper death certificates for the calendar year 2014. The objectives of our study were to document the differences in EHR-sourced death records compared with EDEN-sourced records pertaining to the quantity of information and timeliness. We measured the quantity of information as the number of distinct International Classification of Diseases, Tenth Revision (ICD-10) codes assigned to a death record. Timeliness was measured as the time in hours between a person's time of death as noted on the death record and the date/time stamp of when the record was certified by a physician.

In our analysis, we formed an EDEN/paper group and an HL7 group to support the comparative analysis. The EDEN/paper group included deaths that were completed using EDEN or paper submissions for patients in Intermountain facilities ($n = 1206$). The HL7 group comprised death certificates that were completed using the HL7 EHR interface ($n = 417$).

We examined deaths that occurred during our study period (calendar year 2014) for all patients who died at Intermountain facilities. Physicians at each facility had the option of using the HL7 interface or submitting death records directly through the EDEN system or paper copies. We excluded all deaths that were not due to natural causes. We used cross-tabulations to determine differences in quantity and timeliness between the two groups.

From the information entered by a physician on the death certificate, a total of 10 unique ICD-10 codes may be assigned to each death certificate. One code is assigned as the underlying cause of death and the others are designated as contributing causes of death. Figure 9.1 shows the distribution of the number of causes of death for the HL7 group compared with the EDEN/paper group. As seen in Figure 9.3, greater numbers of ICD-10 codes were listed for deaths reported through the HL7 system compared with the EDEN/paper group.

The peak number of ICD-10 codes reported is higher for HL7 death certificates than for EDEN/paper death certificates. The median numbers of ICD-10 codes on EDEN/paper and HL7 death certificates were four and five,

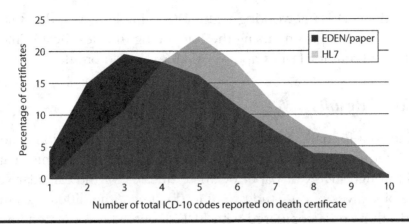

Figure 9.3 Number of unique ICD-10 codes assigned per death certificate by method of certification, Utah deaths September 1, 2013 to August 31, 2014.

respectively. In fact, 42.9% of deaths in the EDEN/paper group listed five or more unique ICD-10 codes, compared with 65.0% of deaths reported in the HL7 system. A Wilcoxon rank-sum test was used to evaluate the difference between the groups. Death records certified in the HL7 system contained significantly more information as measured by the number of ICD-10 codes ($p < .0001$). The results of this analysis have not yet been published.

For this study we calculated timeliness based on the difference between the date and time of death and the date- and time-of-death certification that is stored in the electronic record. Table 9.1 shows the number of death records certified within 72 hours by the method of certification. Timeliness of registration was measured as the number of hours between the date and time of death and the date and time registered. Registration times taking more than 120 hours were considered to be registered in greater than 5 days. Table 9.2 shows the timeliness of registration by certification method. The percentage of death certificates certified through the HL7 system was significantly higher than the percentage certified through EDEN or paper.

Table 9.1 Timeliness of Certification by Method of Certification

Certification Times	Certification Method	
	EDEN/paper	HL7
Certified ≤72 hours	580 (48.1%)	330 (79.1%)
Certified >72 hours	626 (51.9%)	87 (20.9%)
Totals	1206	417
Chi-square $p < .0001$		

Table 9.2 Timeliness of Registration by Certification Method

Registration Times	*Certification Method*	
	EDEN/paper	*HL7*
Registered ≤ 5 days	827 (68.6%)	340 (81.5%)
Registered > 5 days	379 (31.4%)	77 (18.5%)
Totals	1206	417
Chi-square, $p < .0001$		

Discussion and Conclusions

The traditional death certificate process described previously has always been driven by a funeral director in most of the United States. The funeral director has a de facto responsibility to complete the death certificate prior to disposing of a decedent's remains. When death certificates were paper, this responsibility compelled funeral directors to travel to physicians' offices to seek cause-of-death certification. As paper certificates were replaced by EDRS, funeral directors were often relieved of the need to physically deliver a paper certificate, but still felt the onus of asking a physician to certify the death electronically. In either case, the funeral director's request for death certification rarely fell into a physician's normal workflow.

We hypothesized that our EHR death certificate interface would allow physicians to complete death certification within their workflow, resulting in more timely and relevant death information. For hospital deaths in particular, physicians often complete death certificates within hours of a patient's death and prior to being contacted by a funeral director. Physicians report anecdotally that completing the death certificate within the EHR falls into the workflow of other required tasks when a patient dies, such as writing a death note in the patient's record. Our results show a significant improvement in the timeliness of death certification and registration. It is also reasonable to conclude that the access to a patient's record when completing the death certificate or the shorter time interval between death and death certification, or both, results in an abundance of information reported using the EHR interface. Our study did not specifically address the quality of information reported from the EHR, but such an assessment needs to be completed.

Our study results were presented in a report to the National Association of Chronic Disease Directors (NACDD); however, they have not yet undergone peer review or been published. Our results are limited by the fact that there is an inherent selection bias in the physicians who choose to complete death certificates using the EHR interface. However, the results are extremely encouraging from both administrative and public health perspectives.

References

1. NCHS, Mortality data; 2014. Available from: http://www.cdc.gov/nchs/deaths.htm (accessed July 21, 2015).
2. NCHS, Leading causes of death; 2013. Available from: http://www.cdc.gov/nchs/fastats/leading-causes-of-death.htm.
3. Davis K, Staes C, Duncan J, Igo S, and Facelli JC. Identification of pneumonia and influenza deaths using the death certificate pipeline. *BMC Medical Informatics and Decision Making.* 2012;12(1):37.
4. Misialek JR, Bekwelem W, Chen LY, Loehr LR, Agarwal SK, Soliman EZ, et al. Association of white blood cell count and differential with the incidence of atrial fibrillation: The Atherosclerosis Risk in Communities (ARIC) study. *PLoS One.* 2015;10(8):e0136219.
5. Clayton PD, Narus SP, Huff SM, Pryor TA, Haug PJ, Larkin T, et al. Building a comprehensive clinical information system from components. The approach at intermountain health care. *Methods of Information in Medicine.* 2003;42(1):1–7.
6. Pryor TA, Gardner RM, Clayton PD, and Warner HR. The HELP system. *Journal of Medical Systems.* 1983;7(2):87–102.
7. Gardner RM, Pryor TA, and Warner HR. The HELP hospital information system: Update 1998. *International Journal of Medical Informatics.* 1999;54(3):169–82.

Appendix

Acronyms

AHIC   American Health Information Community

BFDR-E   Birth and Fetal Death Reporting—Enhanced

CDA   Clinical Document Architecture

CDA R2   Clinical Document Architecture, Release 2

CGS   Child Growth Summary

DHHS   Department of Health and Human Services

EBRS   Electronic birth registration system

EDRS   Electronic death registration system

EHR-S   Electronic health record system

EHR-S FM   Electronic Health Records System Functional Model

EHR WG   Electronic Health Record Work Group

EVRS   Electronic vital registration system

HBS   Health at Birth Summary

HIT   Health information technology

HITSP   Healthcare Information Technology Standards Panel

HL7   Health Level Seven International

IHE   Integrating the Healthcare Enterprise

IS   Interoperability Specification

ITI	Information technology infrastructure
LDS-VR	Labor and Delivery Summary for Vital Records
LOINC	Logical Observation Identifiers Names and Codes
NAPHSIS	National Association for Public Health Statistics and Information Systems
NCHS	National Center for Health Statistics
NVSS	National Vital Statistics System
MoVERS	Model Vital Events Registration System
PHDSC	Public Health Data Standards Consortium
PHFP	Public Health Functional Profile
PHIN VS	Public Health Information Network Vocabulary System
PHIN VADS	Public Health Information Network Vocabulary Access and Distribution System
QRPH	Quality, Research, and Public Health
RFD	Retrieve Form for Data Capture
SDO	Standards development organization
SNOMED	Systematized Nomenclature of Medicine
VR	Vital records
VR DAM	Vital Records Domain Analysis Model
VRDR	Vital Records Death Reporting
VSCP	Vital Statistics Cooperative Program
VRFP	Vital Records Functional Profile

Index